A WRITER'S GUIDE TO MEDICINE

VOLUME 1: SETTING & CHARACTER

NATALIE DALE, MD.

A Writer's Guide to Medicine
Copyright © 2021 by Ranunculus Press. All rights reserved.
First Edition: November 2021

ISBN: 979-8985420111

Cover and Formatting: Streetlight Graphics

No part of this book may be reproduced, scanned, or distributed in any printed or electronic form without permission. Please do not participate in or encourage piracy of copyrighted materials in violation of the author's rights. Thank you for respecting the hard work of this author.

TABLE OF CONTENTS

Acknowledgments ... 1

Introduction ... 3

Part 1: Setting ... 7
   1. Emergency Department (ED) ... 9
   2. Trauma Center ... 14
   3. Surgical Suite ... 20
   4. Hospital Floors ... 25
   5. Intensive Care Unit (ICU) ... 32
   6. Outpatient Medicine ... 36
   7. Other Settings ... 45

Part 2: Character ... 55
   8. Physicians ... 57
   9. Nurses ... 65
   10. Advanced Practice Providers (APPs) ... 70
   11. Emergency Medical Service (EMS) Providers ... 75
   12. Other Healthcare Personnel ... 80

Part 3: Medicine Basics ... 87
   13. Approach to an Emergency ... 89
   14. Shock ... 96
   15. Cardiopulmonary Resuscitation (CPR) ... 102
   16. Abuse ... 111
   17. Drugs & Addiction ... 123
   18. Environmental Emergencies ... 142
   19. Consciousness & Coma ... 159
   20. Ventilators ... 171
   21. Death & Dying ... 177

Part 4: Q&A ... 187
   The Top 10 Questions I get from Writers ... 189

Appendix 1: Parts of a Hospital ... 203

Appendix 2: Medical Equipment 101 205
Appendix 3: Medical Lexicon 215
Glossary 221
Index 233
Works Cited 248

ACKNOWLEDGMENTS

I**F IT TAKES A VILLAGE** to raise a child, it takes a multidisciplinary team to write a book about medicine (you'll get the joke later, I promise). There are so many people who have helped me on this journey, so many who have supported me from the book's inception to its final copy edit. I couldn't have done it without you, so here are a few shoutouts.

First, to my critique group partners and beta readers: Gary Baysinger, Warren Bull, Jessica Curtis, Mike Davis, Marilynne Eichinger, James Elstad, Warren Friedland, Lisa Hurley, Kalinda Little, Jim Martin, Jennie Miller, Dave More, Elli Rossi, Austin Schock, and Jamie Smith. You not only helped me polish my writing but helped push me out of my comfort zone to get this book out into the world.

Second, to my Rubies–Clare Barnett, Nita Collins, Lidija Hilje, Margaret Johnson, Gisele Lewis, Kristi Rhodes, and Elise Schiller–who acted as my cheerleaders, marketing advisors, and idea sounding boards.

Third, to my doctor friends–Alisha Crowley, Dan Feng, and Sophie Li–who helped make sure I always knew what I was talking about. Special thanks also to all the professionals I interviewed along the way–Concerts Defusco, Heather Farmer, Amy McCarthy, Ryan Ollier, Aletta Vermeulen, and Janettha Vermeulen–for teaching me about aspects of medicine I'd never really considered before writing this book.

Fourth, to all the professionals who helped make this book happen: my editor, Haley Paskalides, for helping narrow this book's incredibly outsized topic, Glendon Haddix for the beautiful formatting and cover design, and Jim Martin for walking the world's most technologically incompetent Millennial through the process of self-publishing.

Finally, a big thanks to my family. To my parents, Jeannette Ellis and Russ Grattan, for their unending love and support, even when I announced I was leaving medicine for a lucrative career as an unemployed writer. To my mother-in-law, Karen Dale, for letting me pick her brain about nursing. And finally, to my husband, Eddy. I can't even begin to count the ways you've bolstered, boosted, and brightened my life.

Thanks so much to everyone who helped me on this journey. I couldn't have done it without you.

INTRODUCTION

FIRST THINGS FIRST

THIS BOOK IS A WRITER's guide. It is intended to help fiction writers depict modern medicine in the American healthcare system (sorry, Canadians). This book is not:

> This book is not intended as medical advice or guidance.
>
> Seriously.
>
> Don't sue me.

- A substitute for medical advice

- A personal guide to self-diagnosis

- Medical school

- Set in a country that has universal healthcare.

- All-encompassing of every possible, incredibly specific, question you might have about your unique story.

Now that we've gotten that out of the way, let me tell you a little about the book and myself.

ABOUT THE BOOK

The idea for this book came about when a writer friend asked me a medical question about her work in progress. I answered her questions, then another writer's questions, and another's. I joined a Facebook Group dedicated to answering writers' questions about trauma and answered a bunch more questions there. The more questions I answered, three things became clear.

First, writers write about medicine all the time. Your story doesn't have to be set in the hospital or have an MC who is a nurse for medicine to play a role. If your character finds a dead body in the woods, is in a car crash, visits a grandparent in a nursing home, has a mental breakdown, loses a pregnancy, punches someone in the teeth, gets shot, or in any other way becomes ill or injured, your story includes medicine.

Second, this stuff is really hard to research on your own. Without an understanding of the basics, internet research can easily be misleading, imprecise, or straight-up wrong. Dr. Google can only get you so far.

Third, there are lots of stereotypes, cliches, and tropes surrounding medicine. How do writers know which contain a kernel of truth and which are downright absurd?

And so, the *Writer's Guide to Medicine* was born.

ABOUT ME

I am a writer and a non-practicing physician. My short stories and essays are published in *Wyldblood,* the *ReAd White & Blue* anthology, the *National Alliance on Mental Illness,* blog and *Flash Fiction Magazine,* among others. I also run a writer's critique group in Portland, Oregon.

After graduating Alpha Omega Alpha from the Chicago Medical School, I started residency in Neurology at Oregon Health Sciences University. Due to an illness, I had to leave residency but not before passing the final US Medical Licensing Exam.

Hold up. Why would you ever want to read a book about medicine written by someone who didn't even finish residency?

That's a good question. Luckily, I have an equally good answer.

In practice, medicine is all about specialization. After medical school, doctors choose a specialty and spend years training to become experts in that field. Medical education, on the other hand, is all about breadth. Medical students rotate through tons of different specialties so they can get a feel for what each has to offer. During residency, young doctors continue to rotate through a variety of specialties related to their chosen field. I personally have rotated through cardiology, emergency medicine, family medicine, gastroenterology, general surgery, internal medicine, a midwife clinic, neurology, neurosurgery, obstetrics and gynecology, palliative care, physical medicine and rehabilitation, pediatrics, pediatric neurology, pediatric surgery, psychiatry (both inpatient and outpatient), radiology, sleep medicine, and trauma surgery. Before medical school, I trained as an EMT and volunteered on a rural ambulance.

Now, let me be clear—I am not an expert in any of these fields. But I have lived and worked in each of those unique settings. I know the basics. And that's exactly what you need: the basics.

HOW TO USE THIS BOOK

To get the most use out of this book, I'd recommend reading it cover to cover—you never know what pearls you might pick up along the way. But if you want to use it more as a reference, picking and choosing the chapters relevant to your story, I promise I won't be too disappointed.

STRUCTURE

This book is divided into three main sections: Setting, Character, and Medicine Basics. There's also a Q&A section at the back, along with a few appendices, a glossary, and an index.

> Word bubbles like this one provide insider tips, like definitions, slang, and the occasional sarcastic comment.

The first section, Setting, covers potential locations where your story might be set. At the beginning of each Setting chapter is a table of sensory stimuli–sight, sound, touch, smell, and taste–that you can use to set the reader in place. Character, the second section, covers healthcare personnel you might incorporate into your story, including their education, scope of practice, and physical identifiers unique to that profession. The third section, Medical Basics, covers what I believe to be the most important fundamentals of medicine that writers should know, though it is by no means exhaustive. In this section, I start each chapter with a vignette, which is used throughout the chapter to highlight important aspects of that condition.

DEFINITIONS

Unless you're in the healthcare field yourself, there's going to be a lot of new terminology. I try to define every medical term the first time I use it. But if you're jumping around, you may miss these definitions. No worries, you can always find them in the glossary at the back!

> Volume 2: Illness & Injury, will follow this format for its entirety.

SUBSECTION: BREAKING DOWN THE CLICHÉ:

Every chapter includes a *Breaking Down the Cliché* subsection in which I identify and address one (or more!) cliches, stereotypes, or tropes associated with the topic. Each of these sections begins with a short, usually sarcastic, example of the cliché in action.

SUBSECTION: REAL TALK

I take an admittedly light tone throughout this book. Medicine is way too wacky and weird for me to take it too seriously. But in the *Real Talk* subsections, I touch upon the darker, more tragic side of medicine. These sections tackle difficult topics that are rife with misconceptions–misconceptions that writers themselves often propagate. I sincerely hope that you read these sections and take them to heart.

FINAL THOUGHTS

Writers have lots of very specific questions, and I can't possibly answer them all in one paltry book. Medicine is a broad, broad field. This book–*Volume 1: Setting &*

Character–focuses on the basics that all writers should know. In *Volume 2: Illness & Injury* (forthcoming 2022), I will go into much, *much* more detail on specifics relating to trauma, diseases, and disorders. The two books can stand alone, but they complement each other well. I highly encourage you to buy and read them both.

Then again, I'm the author. I have to say that.

PART 1: SETTING

1. EMERGENCY DEPARTMENT (ED)

First, let's get something straight: the Emergency Department is a whole department, not a room. Medical professionals refer to it as the ED. However, the term ER has been popularized in American culture, so it's ok if your character still calls it that—as long as they aren't a healthcare worker.

EDs come in many shapes and sizes. Some are specialized, such as trauma centers or pediatric EDs, while others will take anyone who walks through the door. Since we'll be focusing on Trauma Centers in the next section, here, we'll stick to a general medical ED.

> EDs cannot turn any patients away, due to the Emergency Medical Treatment and Labor Act, or EMTALA.[1]

TRIAGE

Not all ED visits are life-or-death emergencies; in fact, the vast majority are not. For this reason, most trips to the ED start with a visit to the triage nurse, who will assess the severity of your character's illness and categorize them appropriately. If your character arrives by ambulance, they'll skip triage and be taken straight back to a room.

> How a character arrives at the ED says so much about them. Did they call the ambulance for a chest cold? Or did they insist on walking three miles with a knife wound because they couldn't afford a cab, never mind an ambulance.

The triage room is usually small and spare, with just enough room for the nurse's chair, a computer, and a place for the patient and one support person to sit. The triage intake usually takes only a few minutes, but if your character isn't actively dying, they're going to have to wait their turn. On average, patients wait an hour and a half just to be taken to their room.[2]

> EDs blow hot and cold—not only in terms of temperature, but in their level of busyness. EDs can be crowded and chaotic one minute, boring and lifeless the next. It's impossible to predict when an ED will become a madhouse.

A WRITER'S GUIDE TO MEDICINE

Sights	People	Nurses, doctors (ED docs, hospitalists, consulting physicians), patients, security guards, family, technicians, EMTs/paramedics, firemen, police, volunteers, medical transporters, interpreters, religious figures, janitors, students, scribes.
	Furniture	Nurse's station, gurneys, computers/chairs, metal chair beside patient bed, curtains, surgical light over bed, partitions, cement or resin floor, sinks with soap and paper towels, cabinets with medical supplies, 'don't fall' posters, whiteboard with key patient info, blanket warmer, med stations.
	Equipment	EKG cart + EKG wires on chest, ultrasound cart, red call button, IV pole +IV bag, oxygen + nasal cannula or full-face mask, pulse-oximeter, blood pressure cuff.
	Patient	Hospital gown, multiple blankets, IV in elbow or hand, pulse oximeter on finger, BP cuff around arm.
Sounds	Voices	Moans, groans, screams, grunts of pain, crying, hushed conversation, laughter (usually amongst staff), polite conversations, phone conversations.
	Technology	Intercom announcements, instruments beeping, alarms, cell phones ringing, tapping of keyboards, scratchy radio at nurse's station.
	Transport	Clattering gurneys, doors opening and closing, squeaky wheelchairs, rolling beds.
Smells	Cleaning	Bleach, Lysol, hand sanitizer, antiseptic, iodine.
	Other delightful scents	Urine, feces, vomit, blood, sweat, cloying perfume or cologne, dead fish (from certain bacterial infections), greasy food.
Touch	Environment	Temperature swings, too cold or too hot, air blowing from vents.
	Discomfort	Pain (sharp, dull, aching, etc.) of injuries, discomfort at IV site or nasal cannula, cold from medication/saline infusion, tightness of blood pressure cuff, soreness, stiffness, itch they can't reach, swollen legs/hands, wristband chaffing.
	Local	Warm blanket, stiff sheets, cool metal rails.
Taste		Stale vending machine food, greasy or overcooked hospital food, metallic taste in mouth from IV meds or saline infusion.

SETTING

Starkly utilitarian, EDs are designed with function in mind. Often, the department is one big area with a nurse's station at the center. The halls are cluttered with gurneys filled with less seriously ill patients and every spare nook and cranny is filled with neatly organized medical supplies. The doors leading to the ambulance bay are constantly opening and closing as new patients arrive–letting in all sorts of weather.

Above the nurse's station is a whiteboard or television screen with the patients' initials, their reason for coming to the ED, and the doctor and nurse assigned. The charge nurse sits at this desk, overseeing the ED and making sure all personnel know where to go. Around the nurse's station are computers where nurses and doctors jockey to write their notes.

The periphery of the department is patient rooms. Sometimes, these are physical rooms with doors, but more often, they're just curtains walling off a small space barely big enough for a bed and a chair. Above the bed is a monitor, which displays your character's heart rate, breathing rate, blood pressure, blood oxygenation, and– if they're on telemetry–the electrical heart rhythm. A moveable surgical light for emergency procedures hangs from the ceiling and banks of drawers filled with medical equipment line the walls. There is also a whiteboard, with the names of the doctor and nurse assigned to the room, as well as other critical information.

> Telemetry is used for continuous monitoring of heart rhythms. It does not replace EKGs.

The sights, sounds, and smells of an ED can be overwhelming. Patients rolled by on gurneys might have blood gushing from multiple wounds, broken bones sticking out of their skin, or horrifying burns. They might be covered in maggots or feces, screaming at the top of their lungs. Curtained off rooms are hardly soundproof, and your character will be able to hear every moan, groan, and private conversation of the people around them. Worse, they'll be able to smell everything too.

THE EMERGENCY DEPARTMENT TEAM

The ED is filled with a variety of different staff members. Nurses provide most of the hands-on patient care, assisted by nurse's aides and ED technicians. Emergency Medical Technicians (EMTs) and paramedics bring in patients, sometimes accompanied by police and firefighters. Advanced Practitioners, such as Nurse Practitioners (NPs) and Physician

> If your character comes to the ED for a minor injury or illness, they may not see a doctor at all! Instead, they'll be seen by an NP or PA.

Assistants (PAs) see less complicated patients and work in teams with physicians. Respiratory Therapists (RTs) provide breathing treatments, while spiritual leaders (Clergy, Pastors, Rabbi, etc.) speak with family. There are medical transporters pushing gurneys, interpreters speaking in a dizzying array of languages, medical scribes typing as fast as their fingers can fly, and students in short white coats running around grabbing warm blankets for their patients. Pretty much everyone wears scrubs (and during COVID, face masks, face shields, and hair caps), so it can be difficult to tell who's who without looking at their name badges.

Doctors in the ED come in two flavors: ED doctors and consulting doctors. ED doctors specialize in Emergency Medicine and are probably wearing scrubs and a harried expression. Consulting doctors, 'Consults' for those in the know, are specialists called in when a patient has a complicated condition, or if they're going to need admission to the hospital. Unlike the rest of the ED staff, Consults wear business-casual clothes under a long, white coat—unless it's the middle of the night, in which case they're probably wearing scrubs and a scowl for waking them up.

> There is little love lost between ED docs – who generally don't have time to care about mundane details – and internal medicine doctors who thrive on them.

ED providers are accustomed to getting some level of abuse from their patients. After all, they regularly see people who are drunk, high, terrified, or in incredible pain. It is not unusual for an ED provider to have things thrown at them, or even to be sexually or verbally assaulted. And while they try to de-escalate the situation themselves, ED providers rely heavily on security guards, who have more training in de-escalation and restraint.

Because ED providers see patients at their worst, they have a reputation for being jaded. Black humor and less-than-professional language—including some racist and derogatory slang—are everyday occurrences in the ED. Yet many people respond well to this informal approach, appreciating doctors and nurses who can cut to the chase and prioritize the immediate problem at hand.

> Some EDs have police dogs in the department to help keep the peace.

BREAKING DOWN THE CLICHÉ: THE FREQUENT FLYER

Nurse 1: "Oh no."

Nurse 2: "What?"

Nurse 1: "Frank's back."

Nurse 2: *checks the calendar* "Well of, course he is. He's due for a refill of his antifungal toe cream."

Some characters always seem to find their way to the Emergency Department. Literature and television like to poke fun at these ED regulars. Either they're a klutz, a macho-man who keeps picking fights they can't win, or an overdramatic hypochondriac. Either way, the ED and EMS providers groan when they hear the patient's dreaded name.

The thing about this trope is that it's true–to an extent. "Frequent Flyers" are patients who come to the ED so regularly that the providers really do know them by name. However, it's rarely because they can't help toppling off rooftops or picking fights with bullies. Instead, most frequent flyers have chronic medical or mental health conditions for which they are unable to receive appropriate care, often because of a lack of health insurance. Sometimes, they're just cold, hungry, and have nowhere else to go.

2. TRAUMA CENTER

	Trauma Center	Emergency Department
Conditions Treated	Motor Vehicle Collisions (MVCs), traumatic brain/spinal cord injuries, gunshot wounds, stab wounds, serious burns, blunt injuries, multi-organ trauma.	Heart attack, stroke, minor wounds (including broken bones), trouble breathing, abdominal pain, fainting, anaphylactic reactions.
Personnel	Trauma nurses, physicians (trauma surgeons, neurosurgeons, orthopedic surgeons, critical care specialists, anesthesiologists, burn care specialists), nurse anesthetists (CRNAs).	ED Nurses, doctors (ED physicians, hospitalists, consulting specialists), respiratory therapists.
Equipment	Crash cart, FAST ultrasound cart, wound care supplies, Airway cart, procedure cart, portable X-ray, surgical light over bed + regular ED equipment.	EKG cart, Ultrasound cart, red call button, IV pole + IV bag, oxygen + nasal cannula or full-face mask, pulse-oximeter on finger, blood pressure cuff.
Patient	Often unconscious: clothes cut off (including underwear), two IVs (one in each arm) C-collar, backboard, visibly bloody or wounded, new sutures ("stitches"), iodine stain around suture sites.	Usually conscious: hospital gown, multiple blankets, IV in elbow or hand, pulse oximeter on finger, BP cuff around arm.

TRAUMA—AT LEAST FROM A MEDICAL perspective—is any injury or set of injuries caused by an extrinsic agent. Car accidents, burns, stab wounds, gunshot wounds (GSWs), broken bones, concussions, and severed spinal cords are just a few of the types of injuries that fall under the category of trauma. These types of traumatic injuries are unique in medicine for a few reasons. First, they tend to cluster, impacting multiple organ systems. For example, if your character was in a car accident, they might have a broken leg, a shattered spleen, a brain bleed, and several lacerations. Second, traumatic injuries take a long time to heal; your character will need many specialists to help them recover. Enter the trauma team.

TRAUMA TEAM

The trauma team isn't just made up of doctors; it's a multidisciplinary team of specialists. Members include (but are not limited to) trauma, orthopedic, and general surgeons, ER and ICU physicians, anesthesiologists and CRNAs, surgical and ED nurses, radiology technicians, respiratory therapists, and social workers. Depending on the types of

> In the OR, multiple different types of surgeons might be working on your character at once!

injuries your character has incurred, they may also be seen by vascular surgeons, neurologists and neurosurgeons, pediatric surgeons, ophthalmologists, urologists, ear nose and throat doctors (also called otolaryngologists), maxillofacial surgeons, and obstetrician-gynecologists. As your character heals, the team will expand to include rehabilitation doctors (called *physiatrists*) and nurses, plastic surgeons, and physical, speech, and occupational therapists.

Because major traumas require such a large and highly specialized team, many hospitals are not prepared to deal with them. That's where trauma centers come in.

TRAUMA CENTERS

Trauma Centers are hospitals with the capacity and resources to care for trauma patients. There are four levels of Trauma Centers. Since hospitals designated Level III & IV have limited capacity to care for trauma patients, most trauma victims receive care at Level II Trauma Centers–urban community hospitals with experienced general surgeons on-call 24-7.[1] But if

> Uncomplicated traumas, such as broken bones, can easily be cared for at rural (Level III-IV) hospitals.

your character has major multi-organ trauma, they will need a Level 1 Trauma Center.

Level 1 Trauma Centers are equipped to handle the most complicated traumas. They are usually major urban hospitals, with surgeons and ICU specialists in-house 24-7. Level 1 Trauma Centers have extensive trauma support networks, including in-house blood banks, labs, and rehabilitation facilities.

If your character experiences a major multiorgan or life-threatening trauma, they will be transferred to a

> The decision to transfer a patient is always complicated, and surgeon egos sometimes come into play. IRL, this can lead to serious medical mismanagement. In your writing, it can be a tense plot point!

Level 1 Trauma Center as soon as they are stable enough to move. Depending on where your story is set, this transfer could mean anything from a 10-minute ambulance ride to a life flight across state borders.

TRAUMATIC INJURIES

MECHANISMS OF INJURY

Trauma is grouped into two main mechanisms: blunt trauma or penetrating trauma. A penetrating injury is anything that pierces the skin: knives, bullets, shrapnel, even fragments of wood, metal, or bone–if you can imagine it cutting through your character's body, you can use it. Blunt injuries are caused by the force of impact. Types of blunt injuries include crush injuries, falls, acceleration/deceleration injuries, compression, and blunt weapons such as clubs.

Gunshot wounds–GSWs to those in the know–are an unpredictable way to injure your character. Bullets cause not only penetrating injuries but also can create a shock wave that propagates through the surrounding tissue, causing damage far from the bullet's path. GSWs also cause cavitation, a temporary cavity that forms around the bullet as it travels, which can suck clothing or debris into the wound. If the bullet hits bone, it can cause secondary missiles, as bony shards shoot out from the point of impact.

> Not all guns (or bullets) are made equal. If you're going to shoot your character, make sure you know what type of gun (and bullet) they were hit with, and from what range. A hunting rifle is going to do a lot more damage than a handgun.

WOUNDS

There are many types of wounds you can bestow upon your character. These include:

Abrasion: An abrasion is when the superficial skin is scraped away, revealing red, raw skin beneath. Examples include skinned knees and road rash.

Avulsion: An avulsion is when tissue such as skin, ligaments, tendons, or muscle is ripped away from the underlying structures.

> Scalping is a form of avulsion injury.

Contusion: A fancy name for a bruise, contusions are caused by crushed tissue causing bleeding from the tiny blood vessels called capillaries.

Dislocation: When a joint pops out of its socket. Dislocations happen most frequently in free-standing joints, such as the finger, elbow, shoulder, knee, and ankle.

Fracture: Fractures (broken bones) come in three main flavors: stable, open (or compound), and comminuted.

> Greenstick fractures are seen in children.

- Stable fractures, mean the broken ends of the bone line up nicely.

- Compound fractures occur when bone breaks through skin.

- Comminuted fractures occur when the bone has shattered in three or more places.

Hematoma: A hematoma is pooled blood. It can collect in skin, muscle, or even organ tissue.

Sprain: A sprain is the injury of the ligaments, most commonly seen in ankles and wrists.

TREATING TRAUMA

APPROACHING TRAUMA VICTIMS

The first step in the treatment of trauma patients is the Preliminary Survey: ensure the airway is open, check to make sure the victim is breathing on their own, check for a pulse and stop any major sources of bleeding, then look for hidden injuries by testing for neck soreness, making sure the victim's eyes dilate normally, looking for chest wounds, and pressing on the abdomen to elicit pain.

> For more on the Preliminary Survey, check out the ABCs in Ch. 13.

The second step is resuscitation, the immediate steps needed to keep your character from dying. This step includes placing a ginormous needle in each arm and running IV fluids as fast as possible, while simultaneously drawing labs to check their blood type, in case they need a blood transfusion. They'll get a catheter shoved up their urethra to help them pee, and a nasogastric (NG tube) shoved down their throat to suction out the contents of their stomach so they don't throw up. Doctors might even thread an instrument through an artery down to the heart to measure their blood pressures.

> Ever wonder why doctors shine lights in their patients' eyes? It's to look at their pupils, as dilated, uneven, or non-reactive pupils can be a sign of impending brain herniation.

Sometimes, an important aspect of resuscitation is surgery; some wounds can only be treated operatively. Most of the time, these life-saving surgeries are designed to staunch massive blood loss and are performed in the controlled environment of the Operating Room (OR).

The most dramatic form of resuscitation is the Resuscitative Thoracotomy, also called a Trauma Thoracotomy. Indicated only after your character's heart has stopped due to severe chest injury, this procedure is performed in the ED itself.[2] The surgeon cuts open the chest and saws through the ribs just left of the breastbone, cracking open your character's chest so the surgeon can directly access the heart and aorta.[2] It's an impressive procedure that is only performed in the direst situations.

> "Cracking the chest" is slang for an open thoracotomy, where your character's heart and lungs are exposed to the air. It's a dangerous procedure but can be lifesaving.

Once the life-threatening injuries have been addressed, it's time for the third stage of approach: the secondary survey. In this step, the doctor will go back over your character, evaluating them more thoroughly. They'll get X-rays of the chest, neck, and pelvis, searching for hidden fractures, and an ultrasound looking for signs of bleeding in the abdomen. Only once they're sure your character is stable will the trauma doctors care for your character's specific, non-life-threatening injuries, including caring for non-life-threatening wounds.

Wound care starts by examining the wound and pulling out any large debris such as gravel or chunks of asphalt. Then, the wound is flushed with sterile water, a procedure called wound irrigation. Lidocaine shots around the edges of the wound are used to control both pain and bleeding during irrigation. Only after the wound has been properly cleansed it be stapled or sutured shut.

> The medical term for deciding where a patient goes next is **Disposition**, but most medical providers just call it "Dispo."

Suturing, colloquially known as "getting stitches," is a precise technique that uses a thin, curved needle and thread to loosely bring the cut edges of the skin together so that they can heal. Suturing helps control bleeding, promote healing, and reduce scarring. Stapling the wound shut is faster and has lower rates of infection, but because they leave bigger scars, staples are not used on the face, neck, or hands.

Once your character has stabilized, they'll either be discharged home or admitted to the hospital.

BREAKING DOWN THE CLICHÉ: PSYCHOLOGICAL TRAUMA

"Popular Patty needs to be admitted for major trauma, stat!"

"What's the mechanism of injury?"

"The girls at school made fun of her bangs!"

Psychological trauma is very real and can cause a whole host of issues (not just PTSD!). But a trauma center deals with injuries caused by an external agent (blunt force, bullets, heat, etc.), not psychological trauma. And while a major traumatic injury can certainly cause psychological trauma (including PTSD), trauma surgeons aren't going to care one fig about your character's mental state. They'll fix whatever is physically injured, then pawn your character off to a psychologist or psychiatrist to deal with the emotional repercussions.

> PTSD = Post Traumatic Stress Disorder

3. SURGICAL SUITE

The surgical suite encompasses the three settings your character will pass through on their way to surgery: the Preoperative Area (Pre-op), the Operating Room or Operating Theater (OR), and the Post-Anesthesia Care Unit (PACU).

PRE-OP

Sights	**Staff**	Pre-op nurses, surgeons, anesthetists, CRNAs, surgical nurses. All wearing scrubs and hairnets or scrub caps.
	Patients	Well-looking, chatting with friend/family member who accompanied them. Wearing hospital gown, BP cuff, pen marks on skin.
	Equipment	Carts with supplies, IVs/IV start kits, oxygen.
Sounds		Conversations, rolling beds. The one place in the hospital where there aren't machines beeping incessantly.
Smells		Chlorhexidine prep, clean/washed human.
Touch		IV needle in arm, warm blankets, hospital bed, pen on skin as surgeon marks the surgical site

Pre-op is where patients are prepared for surgery. If your character has a day surgery, they'll start here. They'll change into a hospital gown and surgical cap, remove their jewelry, and answer a stream of questions from a seemingly endless parade of healthcare providers. The anesthesiologist will come by to look in their mouth and confirm their medication history, the surgeon will explain the surgery and mark the surgical site with a felt-tip pen, and the pre-op nurse will ask your character to fill out paperwork and answer any questions. By the end of it all, your character might feel ready for an anesthesia-induced nap.

If your character needs surgery, they'll enter the OR on a wheeled bed or gurney, usually pushed by the anesthesiologist or surgical nurse. Rolling into an OR for the first time is a little like stepping into an alien world. While the strange equipment and hyper-sterile environment certainly contribute, the overabundance of people wearing blue, their faces and hair covered, can be disconcerting.

THE OPERATING ROOM

Sights	Scrubbed-in Staff	Wearing blue paper gowns with surgical scrubs underneath, blue masks, hairnets and shoe covers, tan surgical gloves. Hands clasped in front of them (patient awake), placed on blue drapes covering patient (patient asleep), or holding surgical tools.
	Other Staff	Blue or light green scrubs and hairnets/scrub caps, long-sleeved blue shirt over scrubs, rubber clogs or tennis shoes.
	Patient (awake)	Hospital gown, IV in arm, hair cap, ID bracelet. No jewelry or underwear. May look woozy or nervous.
	Patient (asleep)	Naked, covered with blue surgical drapes, only surgical sites exposed. Positioned with bolsters and Bair huggers, surgical site shaved, urinary catheter placed.
	Equipment	Surgical table with foot pedals to position head/feet, bright surgical lights above table with handles covered in plastic, bovie machine, surgical tools (scalpel, forceps, hemostat, etc.), anesthesia gas machine, intubation equipment, patient monitor, IV, Bair huggers, steel table with blue drape set up with instruments in neat rows, steel bucket lined with red biohazard bag.
Sound	Before surgery	Beeping of patient monitor, conversation, clink of tools as scrub nurse counts aloud. Music (soft). Nurse calling "timeout."
	During surgery	Music (blasting), buzz of bovie, whoosh of anesthesia gas machine, soft conversation between surgeon and assists, clack of keys as circulating nurse types.
Smells	Before surgery	Clean. Antiseptic surgical scrub. Sweet anesthesia gas just before going under.
	During surgery	Cauterized flesh, blood. Feces, pus, or gangrene
Touch		Cold room. Cold, hard surgical table, warm blanket, discomfort of IV or strange positioning. Anesthesia mask around face. Cold IV infusion. Woozy/sleepy feeling as anesthesia hits.

If your character is conscious, he'll be met by the staff that won't be scrubbing in to the surgery,

For more on Nurse Anesthetists, see Ch. 10

A WRITER'S GUIDE TO MEDICINE

including the anesthesiologist (or nurse anesthetist), the circulating nurse, and the scrub tech. They'll help your character onto the surgical table–a narrow metal table in the center of the room, covered by a thin plastic mattress– cover him with a warm blanket, and position him comfortably. Your character will be grateful for that blanket: ORs are kept at around 70-degrees. The surgeons and other scrubbed-in personnel will be sweating at this temperature, but your character–dressed only in a thin hospital gown–will get quite chilly.

Once your character is positioned and comfortable, the anesthesiologist will start the anesthesia–either gas delivered by facemask or with an IV infusion–and your character will count backward from ten until he falls unconscious.

> In Level 1 Trauma Centers, the trauma surgeon, surgery residents, and medical students will all scrub in, resulting in a very crowded table.

Once asleep, the OR becomes a flurry of activity. Your character is intubated by the anesthesiologist and placed on a breathing machine. His gown and blanket are removed, and he is positioned for the procedure. The surgical area is cleansed with a chlorhexidine solution, then your character is draped with blue surgical drapes, leaving only the surgical site exposed.

While all this is happening, the rest of the surgical team scrubs in. Scrubbing is a specific procedure designed to maintain a sterile field. Briefly, anyone who is scrubbing in will remove their jewelry, then scrub from their fingertips down to their elbows, keeping their hands vertical so that the dirty water drips downwards. Then, still holding their hands up in a gesture of surrender, they'll walk backward into the OR– pushing open the door with their back–where they'll be met with the scrub nurse, who will help them don their gown and gloves.

Once dressed, everyone who scrubbed in will approach your character and place their gloved hands on the blue drapes. The surgeon or resident will make the first incision, and the surgery will begin. If anyone touches anything other than the

> Breaking sterile field is a sure-fire way to get yelled at.

blue drapes or the sterile surgical tools, they've broken sterile field and will need to leave surgery to scrub in all over again.

The atmosphere of the OR depends on the type of procedure, the urgency of the case, and the surgeon. If it's a routine case, there will probably be music playing–I've heard everything from death metal to baroque choral music–and friendly chit-chat. If the case is life-or-death, everyone will be quiet and focused.

> Some people smell different than others.[1] For some, the smell of grilled pork is mouth-wateringly delectable. Others smell more like burnt hair.

While every surgery is unique, there

are a few universally useful instruments. Scalpels cut through tissue, forceps (a fancy name for tweezers) pick up and separate tissue, while retractors hold the incision site open. Blood vessels can be clamped using hemostats, or surgeons can use a bovie–a thin, pencil-like instrument with a metal tip–which uses electricity to burn blood vessels, cauterizing them shut. Bovies are great at stopping the bleeding, but they also make the whole room smell of burnt flesh.

After a successful surgery, your character will be transferred to the Post-Anesthesia Care Unit (PACU) to recover.

POST-ANESTHESIA CARE UNIT (PACU)

Sights	Staff	PACU nurses, anesthesiologist/CRNAs, surgeons, residents, PA/NP, students, possibly a single family member.
	Patients	Asleep or groggy. Wearing hospital gown, BP cuff, pulse oximeter, IV site, urinary catheter, surgical drainage tubes, bandages, etc.
	Equipment	Carts with intubation supplies, patient monitor, BP cuff, pulse oximeter, IV + IV fluids, oxygen tank + face mask or nasal cannula, patient monitor, suction device.
Sounds		Gurgling (asleep), moans and groans (waking up) or raspy voices (awake) of patients, suction, beeping of monitors, low conversation.
Smells		Clean/washed human, stale air of oxygen through face mask.
Touch		Pain at surgical site, scratchy throat, discomfort of urinary catheter, nausea, chills, wound packing, IV needle in arm, warm blankets, hospital bed.

Characters in the PACU are in a vulnerable state. They're still under the influence of the anesthesia, so their breathing and blood pressure need to be monitored carefully.[2] Sometimes, their swallow reflex is impaired, so saliva will pool at the back of their throat, causing a loud gurgling sound. To keep your character from choking, the nurse will suction out the saliva with a vacuum tube like you'd see at the dentist.

When your character wakes up, they'll have a sore throat from the intubation, may feel nauseated, and will likely have some discomfort at the surgical site. Remember the cauterized flesh from the bovie? Your character has not only been sliced open but burned from the inside out. He's going to be a little uncomfortable.

After successful recovery in the PACU, your character will be discharged home (day surgery) or transferred to a surgical recovery floor. If they are not recovering well, they may be sent to the Surgical ICU (SICU).

BREAKING DOWN THE CLICHÉ:

WATCHING THE SURGERY

"Would you like to watch your loved one be cut open and butterflied like a shrimp?"

Having your character's family standing outside the OR, waiting with bated breath as they watch the surgeon operate simply isn't realistic. First, they wouldn't be allowed into the area. Only approved personnel wearing scrubs, scrub caps, and shoe covers are allowed in the hallways surrounding the OR. Personnel don't have to be completely sterile, but they need to minimize the chance that they'll introduce contaminants into the sterile environment.

Second, most ORs don't even have windows, due to privacy concerns. Surgery is incredibly exposing–your character might be buck naked while being prepped for surgery. If ORs had windows, every surgeon, nurse, student, anesthesiologist, and pathologist walking by would get a show. Instead, the door into the OR, usually located in a small vestibule off the main hallway, has a single window where personnel can peek through if they're looking for someone.

Finally, surgery is kind of horrific to watch. Skin flaps are pulled back, blood spurts, gobs of fat are collected in a bucket, and flesh is seared. I've watched and assisted in plenty of surgeries, but I would never, ever, want to see it done to someone I loved.

The only exception to this rule is scheduled cesarean deliveries, or C-sections. In a scheduled C-section, the partner is given scrubs, a scrub cap, and shoe covers. After the soon-to-be-mom has been anesthetized and draped, a curtain is erected just below her breasts to make sure no one can see what's going on down there. Then, the partner is led into the room and told to stand by the mother's head, behind the curtain. When the baby is born, they're carried back to the partner to cut the umbilical cord. Neither Mom nor partner ever gets to see the actual surgical site.

4. HOSPITAL FLOORS

Hospitals are divided into different types of units and floors. Units, like the ICU, offer the highest intensity of inpatient care. Floors, on the other hand, are for patients needing inpatient care, but who aren't quite as critically ill. Some floors can be accessed easily from a central elevator, while others may only be accessed through other wards or by walking through labyrinthine hallways. Even hospital staff sometimes get lost in the maze.

> Many hospitals don't have a 13th floor, the elevator just skips from 12 to 14!

Your character will be sent to a particular floor based on the reason they were admitted to the hospital. There are lots of different types of floors, ranging from Neurology to Orthopedic Surgery. However, most of the time–and particularly in smaller hospitals–your character will simply be sent to a general medical or surgical floor.

> See **Appendix 1** for a comprehensive list of hospital floors and units.

Most wards have the same general structure: nursing stations, physician workrooms, and conference rooms at the center and patient rooms along the periphery. When your character enters the floor, the first thing they'll see is the charge nurse station–a reception area with a bunch of computers and a whiteboard (or computer screen) displaying a list of room numbers and their assigned doctors, nurses, and CNAs. There won't be a patient name on the chart, just initials to protect privacy. The hallways are wide enough to let two hospital beds pass and are lined with sinks and computer stations.

PATIENT ROOMS

Patient rooms come in many shapes and sizes, but the general layout is usually the same. There's an adjustable hospital bed with railings and buttons to adjust the head of the bed and a monitor overhead

> The monitor won't show your character's heart rhythm unless they are connected to Telemetry.

A WRITER'S GUIDE TO MEDICINE

Sights	People	Patients, family, and friends, nurses (Charge Nurse at the front desk, other nurses rushing around the floor), doctors (hospitalists and medical specialties), PAs, NPs, CNAs, phlebotomists, dietitians, transporters, janitors, social workers, chaplains or other religious figures, volunteers, students.
	Furniture	Hospital bed with IV pole, remote for moving bed height/calling nurse, IV infusion bag/pump, IV catheter in hand, patient monitor above bed, television, comfortable chair or couch, flowers/cards on windowsill, variable height table, commode, sink and paper towels (inside every room, and dotted around halls), cabinets with medical supplies, food trays with plastic cover, HIPAA box beside trash can and recycling.
	Equipment	Red/white/black EKG wires on chest, BP cuff, pulse oximeter, IPC device, oxygen through nasal cannula or face mask, IV + fluid bag, urinary drainage bag, colostomy bag, chest tubes + drains, oxygen canister under bed, suction canister, wound care supplies. Gowning area outside room with sink, paper towels, and PPE, including non-latex gloves, gowns, and masks.
	Patient	Wearing hospital gown and ID wristband, either in bed, sitting in chairs in their room, or walking around the floor with their IV pole in tow. May look very ill or quite well.
Sounds	Voices	Calls for "nurse," family conversations, residents presenting during rounds, nurses presenting during huddle
	Technology	Televisions, cell phones ringing, pagers, intercom announcements, beeping alarms, mechanical buzz of bed as patients sit up/lie down, whoosh of IPCs.
Smells		Hand sanitizer, antiseptic, condition-specific smells, such as infection, feces, or urine.
Touch		Cold room, warm blanket, scratchy blanket or hospital gown, cold plastic rails on bed, pain (sharp, dull, aching, etc.), hunger, discomfort at IV site or NG tube, tightness of blood pressure cuff or IPC, dry nostrils from oxygen, soreness, stiffness, or bedsores, itch they can't reach, swollen legs or hands, wristband chaffing.
Tastes	Hospital food	Greasy, stale bread, bologna sandwiches, Jell-O, mashed potatoes, cold salad bar, stale coffee, skim milk in cartons, ginger ale, juice boxes, cheese sticks, vending machine snacks.
	Also hospital food	Steamed vegetables, sweet potato fries, turkey burgers, fish, Starbuck's coffee, stir fry, fancy baked goods, granola bars.

displaying your character's heart rate, breathing rate, and oxygen saturation. Bags of fluid hang from an IV pole at the head of the bed, and there may be a bag of yellow urine attached to the foot of the bed. Long curtains can be pulled around the bed for privacy, and there's almost always a TV mounted on the wall. The TV remote connects to the bed, so your character can adjust the head up and down. It will also have a call button for the nurse, and a red button for emergencies.

Some patient rooms are private, while others are shared. Shared rooms are quickly falling out of fashion due to the risk of infection and cross-contamination. High-income, private hospitals can promise single-occupancy rooms to all their patients while lower-income hospitals often have to make do with double, triple, even six-bed rooms. These cramped quarters make it difficult to maintain privacy, visit with family, or get a good night's rest. How would your character feel if they were stuffed in a too-small-room with roommates who snore and leave the bathroom smelling like a porta-potty at Woodstock?

> In the ED, IVs are placed in the crook of the arm. But on the floor, they're placed in the hand to give your character more freedom of movement.

THE INPATIENT TEAM

Like the ED and the Trauma Center, the medical team on hospital floors is comprised of a variety of different professions. Nurses and CNAs (Certified Nurse Assistants) are the first line of patient care in any hospital, and this multidisciplinary approach is especially true on the floor. Nurses give medications, monitor vitals, transfer patients, and communicate with the patient and family (among many other things). The primary doctors on medical floors are hospitalists—internal medicine doctors who specialize in taking care of hospitalized patients. In some hospitals, your character's primary provider may not even be a doctor; they could be a Nurse Practitioner (NP) or Physician Assistant (PA) working as part of a physician-led team.

> Hospitalists tend to work in blocks–one week on, one week off–so if your character is hospitalized for less than a week, they'll probably see the same doctor for the duration of their stay.

> For more on NPs and PAs, see Ch. 10.

If your character is admitted to a teaching hospital (and most large hospitals are teaching hospitals), they will primarily be cared for by a team of doctors, including an Attending, a Fellow, residents, interns, and medical students.

> Attendings, fellows, residents and interns are all doctors, just in various stages of training.

An **attending** is a doctor who has completed her residency training and is board-certified in her specialty. **Fellows** are doctors who have completed residency but are pursuing further specialty training. A **resident** is a doctor who is in the process of completing residency, while an **intern** is a doctor who recently graduated medical school and is in their first year of residency. A **medical student** is, well, a student, usually in their 3rd or 4th year of medical school. A **Consult** is a physician specialist, called in by the primary team to provide additional insight. On the medicine floors, commonly consulted specialties include cardiology, neurology, pulmonology, infectious disease, and nephrology. "Calling a consult" is an everyday occurrence, but it can sometimes lead to bruised egos and poor communication. It's an opportunity for intercharacter conflict that can have some very real, and possibly devastating, fallout for your character.

> Doctors wear long white coats–but so do PAs, NPs, and pharmacists. Your character can no longer assume someone is a doctor by the color of their coat.

MEDICAL ROUNDS

If your character is hospitalized, they're going to be rounded on. In a community hospital, "rounding" just means that someone from their primary team will drop by each morning to ask how they're doing and give your character a quick physical exam. But if your character is admitted to a teaching hospital, the process of rounding is going to be quite a bit more involved.

It starts with pre-rounds by the medical students and residents. Since most teams start work rounds at 7 am, pre-rounds start around 6:30 or earlier, if the medical student is particularly green or ambitious. Medical students are assigned patients to care for, but since they have no idea what they're doing, the residents also have to check in on those patients during their own pre-rounds. This system of pre-rounding means your character gets woken up twice–and that's *after* being woken up every two to four hours by the night nurse. If your character thought they were going to get a good night's sleep at the hospital, they were sorely mistaken.

After pre-rounding, the residents and medical students gather in the team room for 'paper rounds,' the preliminary discussion of each patient. This discussion is where a lot of teaching happens, but unless your character is a doctor, they won't be privy to this conversation.

After paper rounds come the attending rounds, wherein the whole team parades from room to room, trailing after the attending like ducklings. At each room, the intern or medical student "presents" their

> How does your character feel about being surrounded by a group of doctors talking about them as if they weren't there?

patient—rattling off your character's key information in rapid-fire speech. After the presentation, the Attending may speak with your character, asking if they have any concerns or questions. And then, the pimping starts.

Pimping is a time-honored tradition of teaching rounds. The attending shoots rapid-fire medical questions at the medical students, who jump down each other's throats trying to answer first. Meant as a teaching exercise, 'getting pimped' can be a brutal experience. As your character watches this drama unfold before them, what are they thinking? Do they feel bad for the poor medical students? Or are they just annoyed that they're missing out on their favorite rerun of MASH?

> While the Attending pimps, the residents and interns are constantly being paged or pulled from the room by nurses.

HOSPITAL FOOD

Diet is an important aspect of a hospital stay. Depending on your character's medical conditions, they may be given a low sodium, low fat, or low sugar diet. Skim milk, lean meats, and sugar-free desserts coming right up!

> Patients who can't eat get an NG tube–a delightful little tube threaded down through your character's nostril and into their stomach so that food and medications can be delivered directly.

Most hospitals have a cafeteria that is open 24-hours, though in the wee hours of the morning, all your character will be able to buy might be a plastic-wrapped ham sandwich and coffee from a machine. However, during the day there are usually lots of options for food. Many hospitals have coffee shops with prepackaged salads and freshly baked goods, or gift shops selling fruit and healthy packaged snacks. Some even have food carts that set up in nearby courtyards and parking lots during the lunch rush. In other words, food options at hospitals are no longer limited to mystery meat and Jell-O.

> Smaller hospitals may be limited to a single cafeteria whose only 24-hour option is a vending machine.

VISITING THE HOSPITAL

Visitors are common on hospital floors. Many hospitals no longer have or enforce visiting hours, though ICUs may have stricter regulations. Friends and family are an important part of healing, and most hospitals allow as many visitors as the patient would like. In fact, hospitals

> During COVID, visitor allowances changed significantly, even for those admitted for non-COVID reasons. Many wards didn't allow any visitors, while others enacted strict requirements. Even delivery rooms often allowed only a single support person.

are legally required to have a support person in the room for people with dementia and other disabilities. Potential visitors simply enter the ward and ask the nurse at the front desk for the patient's room number. The exception to the rule is pediatric floors, which have much stricter identification requirements for visiting children and infants; no one wants kids getting abducted!

Some areas of the hospital have limits on who can visit and what they can bring. Children and those with flu-like symptoms are not allowed in most ICUs. Inpatient psychiatric units have strict limits on visiting hours and the number of visitors, as well as specific procedures for entering the Visitation Room. On the floors, visitors cannot bring fresh flowers, fruit, or plants, as they pose an infection risk. However, most hospitals have an in-house florist, where visitors can send flowers to pre-approved rooms.

BREAKING DOWN A CLICHÉ: THE HIPAA HURDLE

"I'm sorry, I can only tell you whether or not your loved one is dying unless you are family."

HIPAA, the Healthcare Insurance Portability & Accountability Act, is used in film, television, and literature to cover all manner of sins, most notably, the refusal of healthcare professionals to reveal any relevant health information to anyone who isn't family. But that's not really what it's there for.

HIPAA was created in 1996 to protect the sensitive health information of patients as healthcare systems switched to digital health records[1] It requires healthcare providers to take reasonable precautions to protect sensitive patient health information, called Protected Health Information, or PHI. It also requires that your character gets to dictate who they want their provider to communicate with, and how much information can be disclosed. HIPAA doesn't differentiate between friends and family; if conscious, the patient gets to make that decision on a case-by-case basis.

> Medical professionals must dispose of PHI in locked HIPAA boxes. But beware; once something goes in a HIPAA box, it never comes out! Is it just me, or does that sound like a fun plot point?

If your character is unconscious, providers can reveal medical information to friends or family if, in their professional judgment, they believe it will be best for your character. Often, this decision means revealing PHI to someone who will make healthcare decisions for your unconscious character. And they need not be family. A medical professional can reveal PHI to a

> PHI regarding mental illness, addiction, and STIs have additional layers of protection.

partner or a good friend just as easily as they could if it were a blood relative. Often, it's a simple matter of who is present.

There are a lot of nuances regarding the choosing of surrogates for medical decision-making, but that's way beyond the scope of this book. For now, just let me say that if your character has a close personal relationship with someone who is unconscious and hospitalized, no medical professional should blow them off simply because they aren't family–the key word being *should*. Medical professionals are human and are subject to all the racist, sexist, classist, homophobic, and patriarchal biases as the rest of us. If your story needs a doctor that refuses to release PHI to non-family members, it isn't unreasonable for that to happen, especially if you explore that character's underlying biases and reasons for refusing such a reasonable request.

> There are times when it is appropriate to refuse to release an unconscious character's PHI to anyone – including family. This is particularly important when abuse is suspected.

5. INTENSIVE CARE UNIT (ICU)

At first glance, ICUs can seem like hopeless places, with patients immobilized and hooked up to machines, their families huddled beside the bedside. Many that end up in the ICU will die. Yet, most will not. Somewhere between 81-92% of patients survive their ICU stay.[1] These patients are the sickest, frailest, most unstable patients in the hospital, yet most of them survive. I find that incredibly heartening.

SETTING

ICUs are full of a variety of strange and alien-looking equipment: ventilators, EEG monitoring, feeding tubes, ECMO machines, and more. Like on the floors, there will be a whiteboard on the wall with the names of the assigned nurse and doctor, as well as pertinent medical information such as diet and pain level. Not every patient needs every piece of equipment, but ICU rooms need to have everything readily available in case a patient crumps or crashes. This Boy Scout level of preparedness leads to rooms crammed with equipment, with machines and wires and tubes seemingly going everywhere at once. For the uninitiated, it can feel overwhelming.

> "Crumping" is medical slang for a patient who is getting worse quickly. "Crashing" is slang for a patient that is actively trying to die..

> **ECMO** (Extracorporeal Membrane Oxygenation): colloquially known as a Heart-Lung Machine.
>
> **EEG** (Electroencephalogram) monitors brain activity and seizures

> All Pediatric ICUs (PICUs) and Neonatal ICUs (NICUs) will be locked units due to the danger of kidnapping.

ICUs are often locked wards, so anyone wanting to come in will need either an access card or will need to be buzzed in by the ICU Charge nurse. This protective measure prevents unwitting families from wandering in during distressing interventions and can also protect patients from unwanted visitors. Urban trauma centers, especially

Sights	People	Patients, family (1-2 only), nurses in scrubs, doctors in scrubs & white coats (intensivists), PAs and NPs, RTs, SLPs, chaplains & other religious figures, janitor.
	Furniture	Single rooms with glass doors, ICU beds with pressure-relieving mattress and IV pole, single metal chair beside bed, photos and cards hanging on wall, nurse's station with computers, physician team room, waiting area with easy-to-clean chairs, end tables, and television mounted on wall.
	Equipment	Non-latex gloves, gowns, masks, shoe covers, and other PPE outside room (for isolation), oxygen canister under bed, COWs/WOWs.
	Patient	Often unconscious, sedated and/or on ventilator, wearing hospital gown, wires/electrodes on chest, blood pressure cuff, pulse oximeter, ID wristband, bandages, IPCs, oxygen through nasal cannula, face mask, or intubation tube, NG tube, IV catheter in both arms, chest tubes, surgical drains with suction canister.
Sounds	Voices	Conversation of rounding ICU teams. Muted conversations of family.
	Technology	Everything beeps: monitors, IV infusion bags, suction lines, ventilators. Whoosh of ventilators, IPCs, and pressure-relieving mattresses. Buzz of doors to unit opening.
Smells		Cleaning and disinfectant, occasional whiffs of infection (C. diff), feces, or urine.
Touch	Patient	Cold room, warm blanket, scratchy blanket or hospital gown, plastic rails on bed, pain (sharp, dull, aching, etc.), hunger, discomfort at IV site, nasal cannula, or NG tube, tightness of BP cuff or IPCs, soreness, stiffness, or bedsores, itch they can't reach, swollen legs or hands, wristband chafing.
	Family	Cold room, hard metal chair, loved one's hand, hunger, discomfort/stiffness from sitting.
Taste	Food	Hospital food, vending machine food.
	Meds	Metallic taste after saline injection, bitter medications.

ones in areas with high rates of gang violence, are more likely to have 'locked' ICUs than sleepy rural hospitals.

The rooms in ICUs generally have glass walls and doors, so that the nurses can keep an eye on their patients from the hallway even when the doors are closed. Curtains can be drawn to protect privacy, but they usually aren't, so if your character is walking (or being rolled) down the hall of an ICU, they'll be able to see the other patients. Most will be unconscious or sleeping, wrapped in bandages and C-collars or hooked up to ventilators. It's enough to make anyone–especially a family member already terrified for their loved one–start to tear up.

While ICU rooms are big enough for several people to move around a patient's bed, when sh*t hits the fan, they can feel Tom-Thumb-Tiny. When a patient is crashing or needs a procedure, medical staff will converge on the room and the family will be shepherded to the ICU waiting room.

The waiting room is usually outside the locked area so that families can wander the hospital while they wait. ICU waiting rooms tend to be some of the quietest, most tension-filled rooms in the hospital, as families wait with bated breath, knowing their loved one could be dying.

THE INTENSIVE CARE TEAM

Patients in ICUs are monitored very closely by a team of healthcare professionals led by a doctor specialized in intensive care, called an intensivist. Unlike floors, ICU rounds tend to be multidisciplinary. This multidisciplinary approach means that, in addition to the attending, residents, interns, and medical students, the rounding team will likely include nurses, pharmacists, case managers or social workers, and respiratory therapists. Sometimes, clergy or religious figures are included, and the patient's family may be invited to weigh in. The result is a mob of people moving slowly from room to room, making it difficult to walk past.

> In the ICU, respiratory therapists monitor and maintain patients on ventilators.

While your character might be overwhelmed by the sheer size of the medical team, one advantage is that your character will get a lot more individualized care and attention. The nurse-to-patient ratio is much smaller in ICUs, often as low as 1:1, and the doctors have fewer patients as well.

> Nurses in the ICU often take notes on WOWs (Workstations on Wheels) or COWs (Computers on Wheels). They're the same thing; a computer on a wheeled cart.

> More on running a Code Blue in Ch. 14: CPR.

ICUs are reserved for the critically

ill. So, once your character is off death's doorstep, they'll be transferred back to the floor.

BREAKING DOWN THE CLICHÉ: CODE BLUE

Hospital PA: "Code Blue, ICU room 469"

All the residents drop what they're doing and race to the room

First one there gets to lead the Code

Everyone else stands in the doorway and sulks

There is definitely some truth to this cliché. When a "Code Blue" is called over the PA system, it means that someone (it doesn't have to be a patient) has stopped breathing, or their heart has stopped–usually both. When that happens, the Code Team really does drop everything and hurry to get to the coding patient. Any medical or nursing students in the area will also flock to the room to wait in line for their chance to practice giving chest compressions. But that's where the similarities stop.

Not every intern, resident, or doctor in the hospital is going to stop what they're doing when a Code is called–that would be madness. Instead, the hospital assigns a "Code Team" who is responsible for responding to any and every Code Blue in the hospital. Team makeup varies by hospital, but in teaching hospitals, it usually rotates daily between the various inpatient medicine teams. At night, the on-call team runs Codes. When a Code is called, the Code Team will politely excuse themselves from whatever they're doing and WALK (no one runs in the hospital) to the room in question, grabbing the Code Cart on the way.

These teams still have their census of patients to care for, still have all their notes to write, but they have the added responsibility of responding to Codes, which–once you add in the extra paperwork–can add hours to a resident's day. Once the initial excitement of running a Code wears off, hearing a Code called overhead is more likely to be met with groans rather than enthusiasm.

While ICUs call more than their fair share of Codes, a Code can happen anywhere in the hospital. I once had to respond to a Code called from the hospital parking garage. If the victim is on hospital premises, and a healthcare provider finds them, they'll call a Code.

> The Code Cart is a wheeled cart full of the supplies needed to run a Code.

6. OUTPATIENT MEDICINE

Outpatient medicine is everything that happens outside the hospital, ranging from a wellness check to imaging and laboratory testing. You're probably familiar with many of these settings–hopefully you've seen your doctor at some point in the last ten years–so I'm going to keep this brief.

CLINIC

You know the drill. Your character checks in with the medical secretary, fills out some paperwork (on a clipboard or a tablet-on-a-stand if they're swanky), then waits until their name is called. The medical assistant takes your character back to the room, takes their vitals, then tells them to wait until the doctor arrives. And it could be a long wait–Primary Care Practitioners (PCPs) are notoriously overscheduled and often run very, very late.

When the PCP arrives, she'll wash her hands, then perform a quick history and physical, asking what brought your character in today. Most PCPs are scheduled for 15 minutes (or less) per patient, which isn't much time if your character comes in with a laundry list of different complaints–the provider might have to repeatedly redirect your character to their most pressing concern, annoying everyone involved. Oh, and she'll probably be typing on the computer the whole time your character is talking; PCPs don't have the luxury of spare time to document each visit, so many of them write their notes as they go.

> **Vital Signs (Ch. 14)**
> - Heart rate
> - Breathing rate
> - Blood pressure
> - Blood oxygen level
>
> Sometimes Includes:
> - Temperature
> - Weight

THE PRIMARY CARE TEAM

Notice how in the above section, I kept saying "PCP" instead of "doctor"? There's a reason for that. Not all PCPs are doctors; as the US healthcare system cuts costs and extends care to a larger population, more and more primary care is performed by non-physician advance practitioners, such as Nurse Practitioners (NPs) and Physician Assistants (PAs).

Sights	People	Specialty doctors or Primary Care Providers (PCPs), Nurses, Medical Assistants (MA), Medical Secretaries, other patients and their families.
	Waiting Room	Front desk, easy-clean chairs, end tables with magazines, signs telling you to cover your cough, clipboard with medical information, pens, Keurig machine, face masks for patients with cough, clock.
	Patient Room	Medical exam table covered by paper, chairs, computer and stool, sink, soap/paper towels, hand sanitizer, cabinets filled with medical equipment, magazines, anatomic models, medical posters, prescription flyers, clock.
	Equipment	PPE, tongue depressors, thermometer, BP cuff, vitals care cart, otoscope and ophthalmoscope, hospital gown, specialty-specific equipment, red sharps & biohazard containers.
Sounds	Waiting Room	Low murmur of voices, children playing, babies crying, MAs calling patients, shuffling feet, squeaking wheelchairs, cell phones, hum of fluorescent lights.
	Patient Room	Crinkle of paper on bed, voices from hallway, knock of doctor/nurse upon entering room, ticking clock.
Touch	Waiting Room	Uncomfortable chairs, solid arm rest, flipping through magazine, warmth of jacket/winter clothes.
	Patient Room	Hot/stuffy vs. overly air-conditioned, hard plastic chairs, stiff gown, uncomfortable pressure of BP cuff, thermometer under tongue, discomfort of exam, jump of muscles from reflex hammer, too-bright light in eyes, cold stethoscope, pressure on abdomen during exam.
Smell		Disinfectant, cleaning (lemon, pine), other people's body odor or perfume.
Taste		Vending machine snacks, Keurig coffee in a paper cup.

Chapter 10 is completely dedicated to Advanced Practitioners, so I'm not going to say too much more here. Just be aware that if your character goes in for a check-up, they're as likely to be seen by an NP or PA as a "real" (please note the air quotes) doctor.

> Most PCPs can treat garden-variety anxiety and depression. Your character will only need to see a psychiatrist if their disease is particularly severe or resistant to treatment.

Dentistry	Dental chair, silver tray with sterilized instruments, posters on ceiling, sunglasses, blue bib, X-ray equipment, buzz of drills, taste of fluoride, discomfort of instruments in mouth, heat of lamp, numb lips/tongue/face.
Dermatology	Poster showing stages of melanoma or other skin cancer, silver tray with sterilized instruments, liquid nitrogen (for warts), blacklight (called Woods Light), discomfort after biopsy or freezing warts off.
Cardiology	Model of heart, posters demonstrating plaque buildup in arteries, EKG cart, cardiac ultrasound machine, whoosh of heartbeat on ultrasound.
Nephrology	Model of genitourinary system (kidneys and bladder).
Neurology	Model/posters of brain, spinal cord, and peripheral nervous system. Pharmaceutical pamphlets. Reflex hammers and tuning forks. Discomfort of reflex and strength testing.
Neurosurgery	Models of spine, skull, and brain. Reflex hammers and tuning forks. Post-surgical care supplies (tape, bandages, suture removal, etc.).
Ob/Gyn	Model of women's reproductive organs, pictures of babies and pregnant women on walls, stirrups on exam table, portable ultrasound machine, whoosh of fetal heartbeat, discomfort of pelvic exam, cold ultrasound gel.
Oncology	Smell of disinfectant. Medication pamphlets, positive message posters, microscope and sample slides.
Ophthalmology	Eye chart, ophthalmoscope, tonometer (air puff into eyes), phoropter (machine with all the gears to determine prescription strength), slit lamp. Sample frames on display in waiting room.
Orthopedic Surgery	Models of hip/knee/elbow joint, suture removal kit, casting supplies, buzz of saw and smell of cut plaster during cast removal.
Pediatrics	Bright decorations on walls and ceiling, posters of famous characters, toys, otoscope/ophthalmoscope. Sounds of children crying or playing, smell of dirty diapers
Physiatry/ Sports Medicine	Instrument trays with injection materials, ultrasound and/or nerve conduction machines on a cart, mini-gym area for physical therapy.
Psychiatry	Comfortable chairs and desk with bookshelves. Looks more like living room than doctor's office. May or may not have a couch.
Pulmonology	Posters of lungs, photos of diseased lungs, posters warning against smoking.
Surgery	Suture removal kit. Model of organs in abdomen. Wound care supplies.

SPECIALTY CLINICS

Sometimes, your character may need to go see a specialist instead of their primary care doctor. They might see an oncologist for their cancer treatment, a psychiatrist for their depression, or a surgeon following up after their recent appendectomy. For the most part, specialty clinics look, feel, and sound just like a regular doctor's office, though some specialties tend to be swankier than others. Once your character gets into the exam room, there will be equipment unique to that specialty, as shown in the (non-exhaustive!) list above.

LAB

Sights	People	Phlebotomists, medical assistants, medical secretary, other patients.
	Furniture	Blood collection chairs, privacy curtain, computer, single-person bathroom with two-way cabinet for placing samples.
	Equipment	Tourniquet, chlorhexidine or alcohol wipe, butterfly needle, plastic tubing, tube holder, vacutainer blood bottles with multicolored tops, urine sample container, patient labels, gloves.
Sounds		Polite conversation, asking for name and birthdate, click of vacutainers as they change out tubes, soft spatter of blood into vacutainers, doors/curtains opening and closing, spatter of urine into cup, kids crying, clack of keyboard.
Touch		Pain of needle prick, tightness of tourniquet, lightheadedness or tingling in hands and feet.
Smells		Cleaning solutions, hand sanitizer, urine or feces (in bathroom).
Taste		Metallic tang (after blood donation or other large blood loss).

Labs can be located inside hospitals, within outpatient clinics, or even in freestanding healthcare settings. The most collected specimen in labs is blood, but almost any human tissue that can be sampled without a surgical procedure can be collected at a lab, including urine, feces, semen, saliva, sweat, sputum (the stuff your character coughs up), and more. Every lab will have a unisex, single-stall bathroom for the collection of samples. Besides the usual toilet and accouterments, these bathrooms will have a small stainless-steel shelf with alcohol wipes and other supplies as well as posters spelling out how to perform a 'Clean Catch' urine

> Since most people can't poop on command, fecal samples are take-home tests.

sample. On one wall, there will be a cabinet to place the sample in, with a door on the opposite side leading to the lab, so technicians can pick up samples without bothering the patient in the restroom.

IMAGING CENTER

Sights	People	Medical secretary, other patients and family, technicians (wearing scrubs), radiology nurse, radiologist (only for procedures).
	Waiting Room	Similar to clinic: easy-to-clean chairs, televisions, signs instructing where to stand.
	Changing Area	Locker for clothes, key to locker with tag or other personalization, laundry hamper, neatly folded scrubs to put on, seat for changing.
	Procedure room	Lead-lined room with no external windows, imaging equipment, glass window looking into separate technician area with computers and paperwork, lead jackets hanging on walls.
Sounds	General	Machine whirring, technician's voice through intercom or headphones, music.
	MRI	Very loud banging, knocking, and beeping.
	Ultrasound	Whoosh of heartbeat.
Touch	General	Cold table, warm blanket, discomfort of lying very still for a long period.
	CT or MRI (with contrast)	Needle prick, cold rushing up arm at IV site, feeling of losing control of bladder.
	Ultrasound	Cold gel, pressure of probe, uncomfortably full bladder.
	Mammogram	Painful pressure on breast.
Smell		Disinfectant, cleaning solutions.
Taste	CT (with contrast)	Metallic tang in mouth.

An imaging center—whether part of a hospital or a free-standing facility—is where your character will go to get all their medical imaging, from simple X-rays to complicated CT-guided procedures. Depending on the type of study your character needs, their experience will be vastly different.

X-RAY

X-rays use a very small amount of radiation to create an image based on the different densities in your body. Looking for differences in density means they are great for imaging bones (high density) and lungs (low density). If your character might have broken a bone or if they have a cough, the first step is almost always an X-ray. The procedure itself takes only minutes; your character is positioned on a table or standing in front of the machine, while the technician moves a moveable arm around them. Then, the technician goes into a lead-lined room, presses the button and they're done. Easy peasy.

COMPUTED TOMOGRAPHY (CT) SCAN

A CT scan is a 3D x-ray that is great for looking at your character's internal organs and blood vessels. CTs are used to look for bleeding, blood clots, tumors, abscesses, and more.

> Medical professionals just call them CTs. The only place you can get a "cat scan" is at the vet!

But getting a CT is quite different from getting an X-ray. The CT scanner looks like a big white donut; your character will have to lay on a cold, narrow table that will slide in and out of the center of that donut. Your character will hear a soft whirring during the exam, but nothing will touch them. The technician will stand behind a lead-lined wall and may give instructions through an intercom. Your character will have to lay very still for the duration of the exam, which can take between 10-30 minutes.

> CTs produce a much higher dose of radiation than X-rays. An abdomen CT produces ~400x more radiation than a chest X-ray.

MAGNETIC RESONANCE IMAGING (MRI)

An MRI uses magnetic fields to generate a detailed 3D image of soft tissue. MRIs are good for looking at joints, muscles, and the brain and spinal cord. MRI machines look a lot like CT scanners; a big white donut with a narrow table sliding in and out of the central hole called the bore. Only, in MRIs, that central hole is much deeper and narrower; depending on the study, your character may need to be fully inside the machine. There isn't much headroom; the average bore is only 60cm[1]–less than the diameter of your average car tire.

> The bore of the MRI is so narrow that obese patients often won't fit. If your character is obese, they may be sent to the zoo for their imaging, much to their mortification.

MRIs are also loud as h*ll; think somewhere between a food processor and a

A WRITER'S GUIDE TO MEDICINE

jet taking off. To protect their ears (and their sanity), your character will wear chunky, noise-canceling headphones that play soothing music of your character's choice. But don't be fooled—it's still going to be loud. And your character will have to stay super, super still for the entirety of the process, which can last up to 90 minutes. If your character is at all anxious or claustrophobic, they're going to have a rough time.

POSITRON EMISSION TOMOGRAPHY (PET) SCAN

The main use of PET scans is to look for cancer, particularly if the doctors are worried that their cancer may have spread. Your character will be injected with a radioactive tracer and then given a specialized CT scan. The radioactivity won't turn them into Spiderman, but it will cause areas of high metabolic activity—like cancer—to light up like Times Square at Christmas. The test takes about two hours and feels very similar to a CT scan; only, your character will be mildly radioactive for about twelve hours afterward.[2] The radiation won't hurt most people, but your character shouldn't hang out with pregnant women or babies until the tracer is out of their system.

ULTRASOUND

Ultrasounds are good for so much more than looking at fetuses—they are also used to image the heart, blood vessels, testicles, uterus, ovaries, abdominal organs, thyroid, and more. They use sound waves to make generalized pictures—the images produced tend to be gray, fuzzy, and difficult to interpret unless you know what you're looking at. To get an ultrasound, your character will have a small probe covered in gel pressed against the part of the body being studied. But not all ultrasounds are external; sometimes to get a better picture, the ultrasound probe needs to be inside the body. That means ultrasounds can be transvaginal (up the vagina), transrectal (up the bum), or transesophageal (down the gullet). And while ultrasounds are generally not painful, no one *likes* having a giant probe shoved up an orifice.

Doppler—named after the famous 'Doppler Effect'—can be added to any ultrasound to quantify blood flow. If your pregnant character is getting an ultrasound, adding Doppler means she'll be able to hear the fetal heartbeat. But Doppler isn't just for fetal ultrasounds—it can be used to evaluate blood flow pretty much anywhere in the body.

BREAKING DOWN THE CLICHÉ: HOUSE CALLS

Knock on door *Door opens to reveal an older man with a black leather bag*

"Doctor! What are you doing here?"

"Oh, I just wanted to check in and see how my favorite patient is doing."

Unfortunately, the days of a doctor showing up at your character's house to check in on them are well and truly gone. Due to cost, time, and litigation, house calls are no longer a financially viable option for the vast majority of doctors. That doesn't mean your character won't have medical professionals visiting their home–it's just unlikely to be a doctor. Below is a list of professionals who routinely make house calls.

Palliative Care: The one time your character might have an actual doctor (or Advanced Practitioner) visiting them in their home is if they are on palliative care, also known as hospice. To be on hospice, your character has to be actively dying, with an expected lifespan of fewer than 6 months. The doctor will visit with your character and their family, making sure they're comfortable and adjusting medications as needed. If your character is on hospice, they're probably on some pretty high doses of opioids and other drugs. Of course, if your character is being seen by hospice, they'll be cared for by a range of professionals on the palliative care team, including a home health nurse.

> For more on hospice and palliative care, see Ch. 7.

Home Health Nurses provide in-home care for your character, ranging from monitoring vitals and administering medications to performing a home safety analysis. The level of involvement of home health nurses varies greatly, ranging from a one-time visit after hospitalization to daily insulin injections. But unless your character is Christopher Reeves, they aren't going to have a 24-7 home health nurse. Instead, they'll have a home health aide.

> To receive 24-7 nursing care, your character must be both severely disabled and fabulously wealthy. Otherwise, they'll need to be admitted to a Skilled Nursing Facility, or SNF (Ch. 7).

Home Health Aides are non-medical caregivers who help with everything from feeding and dressing to bathing and toileting. Your character may need an aide to come as infrequently as once a week to help with groceries or bathing, or they may require 24-7 assistance. Home Health Aides aren't cheap–they still cost around $15-25 per hour–but they're a lot cheaper than a nurse.

> Paying for home care is a struggle for many families. How do you care for a loved one if you still have to go to work?

- **Occupational Therapist:** Because an occupational therapist's job is to help your character relearn how to manage day-to-day activities, one might visit your character's home to help them navigate obstacles like stairs, showers, and toilets.

- **Speech-Language Pathologist (SLP)**: If your character survived a stroke, has trouble swallowing, or if they have a child with language delay, the SLP might visit them in their home. There are lots of benefits to in-home speech therapy, including helping your character to feel safe, providing familiar routines, and eliminating commutes.

7. OTHER SETTINGS

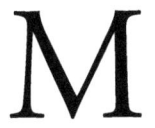

MEDICINE IS NOT LIMITED TO the hospital and clinic. In this section, we'll explore other healthcare facilities where your story might be set.

AMBULANCE

Sights	**People**	Paramedics, EMTs, firefighters, police, bystanders.
	Patient	Street clothes (may be cut off), visible injuries.
	Furniture	Gurney with sheets, pillows, and blanket, narrow bench, shelves filled with neatly organized medical equipment.
	Equipment	Airway equipment (BVM, oxygen, pulse oximeter, suction), cardiac monitoring (defibrillator, stethoscope, BP cuff), radio, C-collar, splints, backboard, PPE, gauze, dressing, tape, emesis basin, patient chart, trauma shears, IV supplies, hand sanitizer, sharps container, needles, syringes, jump bag, reflective jackets.
Sounds		Conversations, moaning/groaning, ambient noise (traffic, television on in the background, etc.), crackling of rig's radio, sirens.
Touch		Weather, uncomfortable gurney, pain, IV site, uncomfortable pressure of BP cuff, thermometer under tongue, discomfort of exam, too-bright light in eyes.
Smell		Disinfectant, cleaning (lemon, pine), body odor, perfume, urine.
Taste		Metallic taste of blood.

While the front seat of an ambulance looks pretty much like a car–though there are a few extra buttons for the lights and sirens–the back is chock-full of medical equipment. The stretcher sits on one side; it has collapsible wheels that allow for easy ingress and

> EMTs don't call the ambulance a bus–it's the rig!

egress. On the other side is a narrow bench where the paramedic–or your character's family member–might sit. The walls of the ambulance are lined with shelves filled with medical supplies, such as bandages and dressings, commercial tourniquets, IV supplies, needles and syringes, glucometer and diabetic testing supplies, intubation equipment, medications, and more.

When EMTs arrive at your character's location, one will grab the jump bag–a sturdy pack full of useful medical supplies–while the other grabs the gurney. They'll hurry over to your character and perform a quick assessment. If your character isn't in immediate danger, they'll take the time to do a thorough exam. But if your character is circling the drain, they'll follow the ABCs to address the immediate, life-threatening issues, then pack your character into the ambulance and use lights and sirens to get to the hospital ASAP.

> ABC's (See Ch. 14)
> A = Airway Protection
> B = Breathing
> C = Circulation

REHABILITATION HOSPITAL

Sights	Staff	Doctors (physiatrist), PAs or NPs, nurses, CNAs, PTs, OTs, speech therapists, clinic managers, dietitians, janitors.
	Patients	Stroke victims, amputees, brain injuries, spinal cord injuries.
	Patient Room	Hospital bed, slings, pulleys, grab bars, wheelchairs, trays, bed enclosure, photos/personal effects. Patient wearing TED hose and nonslip socks, sweat-suits, leg bag around calf (for urine).
	Therapy Room	Walker, stationary bicycle, mats, adapter chair, stairs, practice door, practice car with door, stretch bands, bars, medicine balls, dumbbells walkers, wheelchairs, exoskeleton, heated swimming pool with noodles, weights, and lifts.
Sounds	Patient Room	Alarms (chair alarms, bed alarms, buzzers, etc.), whooshing of IPCs.
	Therapy Room	Conversation, grunts, dropped weights, hesitant footsteps.
Touch		Temperature, uncomfortable chairs, tight IPCs or TED hose, warmth/discomfort of leg bag, tired, difficulty following PT directions, choking, trouble swallowing.
Smell		Disinfectant, cleaning solutions (lemon, pine), other people's body odor or perfume.
Taste		Hospital food, liquid diet, soft diet.

If your character has had a major injury or illness that impacts their ability to care for themselves, they will be sent to a rehabilitation hospital before going home. Sometimes, rehab hospitals are inpatient wings within a larger hospital, other times they are freestanding facilities. Only patients who are medically stable, but still require a high level of daily care, are admitted. Rehabilitation hospitals can provide IV fluids, IV antibiotics, and wound care, but not much more.

A rehab hospital is not a permanent move, but your character will likely spend more time at the rehab facility than they did at the hospital. The purpose of rehabilitation hospitals is to help your character recovery using a variety of different therapies, including physical, speech, and occupational therapy. These therapies can take many shapes. Your character may need to relearn how to walk, speak, feed, dress, or even something as simple as swallow liquids.

> Doctors who specialize in sports medicine and rehabilitation are called physiatrists, or Physical Medicine and Rehabilitation (PM&R) doctors.

Because of their specialized function, rehab hospitals are full of unique equipment meant to maximize your character's abilities. Hoyer slings help patients transfer from the bed to the wheelchair and back again. Bed enclosures prevent patients with brain injuries from falling out of bed. Equipment designed to help with mobility is everywhere, from grab bars by the toilets to walk-in showers. The therapy rooms are covered in soft mats and filled with equipment ranging from simple medicine balls and stretch bands to fake cars and stairs. Not all facilities have pools, but aqua therapy is an important tool many physical therapists use to help their patients get back on their feet. Literally.

> Letter boards are a communication tool for characters with communication barriers. The character simply points to the word, letter, or picture to indicating their desired meaning.

Many different diseases, conditions, and injuries could land your character in the rehabilitation hospital. Some have medical causes, such as strokes, multiple sclerosis, or recent surgeries like hip replacements or amputations. Others, such as spinal cord or brain injuries, are usually due to accidents. Patients at inpatient rehabilitation hospitals can be of any age or gender and need a wide variety of accommodations. If your character needs inpatient rehabilitation, what sort of accommodations might they need?

Days in the rehabilitation hospital are busy, full of a revolving schedule of different therapies. There is rarely downtime, as characters can be

> Not all accidents leading to disability are major traumas. A fall from standing can still cause major injury to the brain or spinal cord.

scheduled for upwards of six different therapies every day. Your character will need to participate in at least two of these therapies for three hours a day, five days a week, to justify their stay at the rehab hospital.[1]

This schedule is exhausting, and it isn't for everyone. Your character may tire out and refuse to participate or he may no longer need the high-level inpatient care. No matter the reason, once your character can no longer participate in therapy, they will be transferred out, either to a skilled nursing facility or back home.

SKILLED NURSING FACILITY & NURSING FACILITY

Sights	Staff	Nurses, CNAs, PTs, OTs, SLPs, dietitians, housekeeping, janitors.
	Patients	Mostly elderly and/or frail. May have feeding tubes, urinary catheters, IV medications, or colostomy bags. Likely needs help walking, feeding, or toileting.
	Patient Room	Hospital bed, slings, grab bars, wheelchair, trays, photos/personal effects, wearing TED hose and nonslip socks, sweat-suits, leg bag around calf (for urine)
Sounds		Alarms (chair alarms, bed alarms, buzzers, etc.), whooshing of IPCs, conversation, televisions.
Touch		Temperature, uncomfortable chairs, tight IPCs or TED hose, warmth/discomfort of leg bag, tired, difficulty following PT directions, choking, lump in throat from trouble swallowing.
Smell		Disinfectant, cleaning solutions, other people's body odor or perfume.
Taste		Hospital food, liquid diet, soft diet.

Nursing Homes and Skilled Nursing Facilities are not the same things, but many people, my own father included, would rather put a bullet in their brain than end up in either one. But what are the differences between them? Do they deserve their reputation?

SKILLED NURSING FACILITIES (SNF)

SNFs are transitional facilities that take care of people who need a high level of nursing–think the kind of round-the-clock care you'd get at the hospital. Nurses work under a supervising

> Skilled nursing facilities are called SNFs (pronounced "sniffs") for short.

physician along with PTs, OTs, and speech therapists. A SNF is very similar to an inpatient rehabilitation hospital; the main difference is that SNFs provide fewer, less intensive therapies.

With an average length of stay of 20-40 days, SNFs are not long-term care facilities.[1] In fact, Medicare will only pay for a maximum of 100 days in a skilled nursing facility.[1] People that need long-term skilled nursing care–such as those reliant on ventilators–have a very expensive road ahead of them.

Like everything in American medicine, SNFs are for-profit facilities, and the quality of care received can vary greatly. While many provide excellent care, some SNFs are notorious for their borderline neglect of their patients. Nonverbal patients sometimes arrive at the ED in poor condition or without an escort to tell the staff what is wrong. SNF patients sometimes arrive with clogged urinary catheters, infected G-tubes, or covered in bedsores. Not all SNFs are this bad, but the poor care provided by some taints the reputation of all.

SNFs are not set up to treat acute medical illnesses. If a person in a SNF gets sick, they're taken to the ER for treatment, usually in an ambulance. But a medical emergency isn't the only reason a person admitted to a SNF might need medical transport. Most doctors no longer do house calls, and that includes visiting SNFs, so if your character needs to see their doctor, they will need to get a ride in a medical transport vehicle.

> Medical transport vehicles transport patients that cannot be moved in a private vehicle. They're usually large, well-marked vans.

NURSING FACILITY

Nursing facilities, also called nursing homes, are long-term care facilities for people who need help with their activities of daily living, such as cooking, eating, bathing, or dressing. Run by LPNs and CNAs practicing under a RN, nursing facilities help people who can't take care of themselves manage chronic health or behavioral conditions. They do not manage complicated medical patients. In other words, if your character is elderly, demented, or otherwise unable to care for themselves, but doesn't need specific medical care, they'll probably need to be in a nursing facility.

> CNA = Certified Nurse's Assistant
>
> LPN = Licensed Practical Nurse
>
> RN = Registered Nurse
>
> See Ch. 9 for more on levels of nursing.

	Skilled Nursing Facility	**Nursing Facility (Nursing Home)**
Staff	Nurses (RN), CNAs, PT, OT, Speech Therapist, dietitian, janitor, maintenance.	Nurses (LPN), CNAs, Dietitians, housekeeping, janitors.
Patients	IV medications, feeding tubes, urinary catheters, ventilators.	Elderly, frail, or bedridden. May have colostomy bag.
Facilities	Private or double rooms, PT/OT area, common room, dining room.	Private or double rooms, living areas, game rooms, dining room.
Equipment	Hospital bed, nightstand, chair, privacy curtain.	Hospital bed, personal clothes in dresser/hanging, blanket and photos from home, chair, privacy curtain.

Nursing homes are not covered by Medicare or most private insurance.[1] And while Medicaid does pay for long-term care, your character will have to meet stringent income requirements to qualify. Besides, many nursing facilities—especially the nice ones—don't accept Medicaid. So, if your character doesn't have long-term care insurance, they're pretty much screwed.

Nursing homes are graded by a federal rating system on a scale from one to five, based on health inspections, staffing, and quality measures. One-star facilities pass the health and safety inspections, but their care is significantly below average. And about ¼ of all nursing homes receive this near failing grade.[2] What does that say about the nursing home industry?

Not all nursing homes are depressing death traps. There are certainly many beautiful, well-appointed nursing facilities that take wonderful care of their patients. But they cost money. Lots of it. How would your character react to being placed in a nursing home? How would they afford it?

> COVID shone a light on the substandard care provided at nursing homes. Understaffing and the for-profit structure led to nearly 100,000 deaths in long-term care facilities between March and November of 2020.[3]

HOSPICE & PALLIATIVE CARE

Palliative care, or hospice, is a team of providers who specialize in end-of-life care. They focus on improving the quality of life, rather than extending its quantity.

PALLIATIVE CARE TEAM

The palliative care team is comprised of several different providers, including doctors and nurses specializing in palliative care, social workers, volunteers, and clergy. The job of the palliative care team is to help manage pain, provide emotional and grief support, and coordinate care.

Hospice is for anyone with a terminal illness who wants to focus on their quality of life. A person can choose hospice at any point if their expected lifespan is less than six months, meaning your character could choose hospice even if they're just minutes from death. Conversely, your character could choose hospice, then live another year. Estimations of life expectancies are not perfect, and your character will not lose their hospice coverage if they don't die within exactly six months.

PALLIATIVE CARE LOCATIONS

Many choose to receive hospice care at home, with a friend or family member acting as their primary caregiver. Your character will get to take their last breaths in their own home, surrounded by the people they love. But, due to cost and the significant burden of 24-7 caregiving placed on your character's loved ones, your character might not be able to choose home hospice. Luckily, there are other options.

Palliative care can also be administered within the hospital or SNF. The hospice team takes over the primary management, but your character doesn't have to move. Another option is a freestanding Hospice House. Intended for people who can't go home, freestanding hospice facilities offer a calming, home-like environment while providing the intensive, 24-hour care needed. Many hospice houses are associated with non-profits and provide care to those who could not otherwise afford these intensive services.

> End of life care is extremely expensive. Luckily, almost everyone qualifies for financial assistance for hospice.

Hospice homes are quiet, reflective places. Families and staff speak in low voices, not wanting to disturb the grief of those around them. They are often bright and sunny, with open windows and pastoral paintings hanging on the walls. Every patient gets a private room, decorated with homey touches that make it feel more like a bedroom, despite the hospital bed. Often, there's a garden with walkways and benches. There's also usually a small chapel or prayer space. Sometimes, there's quiet music or a therapy animal making the rounds. The scent of all the fresh-cut flowers can almost overcome the sharp bite of disinfectant. Almost.

> Your character can bring in anything they want from home–a favorite quilt or pictures of loved ones. Even beloved pets are usually allowed to visit.

HOSPITAL MORGUE

Sights	Staff	Forensic pathologist, medical examiner, coroner, autopsy technicians, crisis counselors, religious figures.
	Patients	Cadavers with toe tags, in black plastic body bags, stainless steel, refrigerated lockers, or naked on exam table.
	Post-mortem Bay	Stainless steel exam table, shelves, rolling buckets, and hanging scale. White or stainless-steel body refrigerators. Draped equipment cart with scalpels, bone saw, forceps, etc. Floor with grates and drains. PPE, biohazard bags.
Sounds		Hum of bone saw, squelch of organs and fluids, music.
Touch		Cold air, cold steel tables, cold flesh, rigid muscles.
Smell		Fritos (from sawed bone dust), blood, feces, necrotic flesh.
Taste		Please don't taste anything in the morgue.

The care of bodies after death is shrouded in mystery. Even when I was practicing, I didn't know what happened to my patients after they died. For most, they go to the hospital morgue, then to a mortuary or cremation center where they are prepared for their final rites. Some, however, require an autopsy, also called a post-mortem exam.

THE POST-MORTEM TEAM

Turns out, it's a bit complicated. Three types of professionals can perform the post-mortem examination: pathologists, medical examiners, and coroners. All three can issue death certificates.

> See Ch. 20 for details on how an autopsy is performed.

A forensic pathologist is a doctor who specializes in the study of human tissue. They usually work in hospitals and perform diagnostic tests to figure out the cause of death, confirm diagnoses, or study tissue. Medical examiners are also doctors (usually forensic pathologists), appointed by the local government to examine bodies and assist police investigations. Because they specialize in toxicology and analyzing a body for violence, medical examiners are often expert witnesses during trials. If you're writing a mystery or thriller, your characters will probably be working closely with a medical examiner.

> For more info on the changing role of autopsies, watch John Oliver's "Last Week Tonight" segment on Death Investigations.[5]

Not all counties in the US use medical examiners;

some rely on coroners instead. Coroners are elected officials. They are not required to have a medical degree and are trained on the job to examine bodies after death. Coroners are rather controversial, given the double whammy of insufficient medical training and the potential conflicts of interest during election cycles.[4] However, rural hospitals are often unable to afford or attract medical examiners, so coroners remain the only option. How would it affect your story if the coroner–the only person who can declare the victim's cause of death–is more interested in getting re-elected than getting to the bottom of the case?

MORTUARIES, FUNERAL HOMES, AND CREMATORIUMS

Morgues are where bodies are stored after they die in a hospital, and where they are examined by autopsy. Mortuaries are where bodies are prepared for their funeral and burial. While morgues are populated by pathologists and pathology assistants, mortuaries employ morticians, also called funeral directors or undertakers. Their job is to prepare the body and assist the family in preparation for the funeral. Morticians may be assisted by mortuary assistants, embalmers, and even cosmetologists, whose job it is to make the cadaver look less dead.

If your character is getting cremated, they'll go to a crematorium. The family will work directly with the Crematorium operator or director, while a crematorium technician will be the one to burn the body. If your character's family wants to watch the cremation, they can–it's called a witnessed cremation–but it's going to be a pretty traumatic experience.

BREAKING DOWN THE CLICHÉ: VISITING THE MORGUE

"I know! Let's go down to the morgue and check out the body ourselves!"

"What a good idea. I hear it's beautiful down there this time of year."

There are two things wrong with this cliché. First, doctors don't go down to the morgue. Like, ever. Except for pathologists. There isn't much to be gained by going down there. Even if the doctor has a question that could be answered on autopsy, a pathologist will perform the autopsy and relay the results to the referring physician. Pathologists are highly trained in the examination of dead bodies–your average-Joe physician (or cop) isn't going to see anything they missed.

The second thing wrong with this cliché is that morgues are not pleasant places. Look at any Crime or Medical TV show and you'll find a clean, brightly lit facility, with the medical examiner wearing jewelry and a neat white coat. This was decidedly not my experience. Hang on to your handkerchiefs, folks, this is about to get gruesome.

> This is only my personal experience, so take this with a grain of salt.

The only time I ever went into a morgue was during medical school when, for a pathology class, I assisted with a post-mortem examination. It was in the basement of the hospital, down a long, poorly lit hallway filled with lockers and spare medical equipment. The morgue was small, just three interconnected rooms. The first room had more lockers and a computer that looked like it was from the early 90s covered with paper files. A sign instructed me to don a protective yellow gown, blue latex gloves, shoe covers, and face shield. I did so, then proceeded to the second room.

As I opened the door, the smell—rotting fruit meets diarrhea—crashed into me. The cadaver was already on the table in the second room, a moveable surgical light illuminating her naked breasts and abdomen. At the head of the bed was a hanging scale with a stainless-steel basket. The shelves lining the room were cluttered with medical-grade scales, red biohazard bags, dissection tools, and plastic containers—like those you might get from a takeout restaurant—filled with preserved organs. There was a stainless-steel sink in one corner, and the room was freezing. The floor was polished cement, though there was a metal grate at the base of the exam table. A cart covered in blue surgical drapes sat on the opposite side of the exam table, covered with dissection equipment set out in neat rows. On my left, I could see the third room, lined with silver doors.

> Autopsy equipment includes the usual surgical tools—scalpels, hemostats, and forceps—alongside stranger tools, like bone saws and shears as big as garden loppers.

The pathologist, already wearing his gown, gloves, mask, and rubber boots, introduced himself then walked me through the external examination of the body. When he made his first Y-shaped incision, I quickly appreciated the utility of the metal grate in the floor, as copious fluids spilled from the body. The smell was overpowering, and we quickly found the source of the stench—a bowel perforation that had slowly been leaking feces into her abdominal cavity. It was the cause of death. When I got home, I threw away every article of clothing I'd been wearing—including my shoes—and took a very long shower.

> To me, sawed bones smell like Fritos.

I've since been told that not all morgues are this grim, not all autopsies this traumatizing. That some really are well-organized and brightly lit. Many autopsies are defined more by the smell of the bone saw than by feces and necrotic flesh. But if you're writing a scene in the morgue, please remember that pathology departments are chronically underfunded; you're much more likely to end up in a smelly, dimly lit morgue than a shiny one.

PART 2: CHARACTER

8. PHYSICIANS

Credentials: MD (Medical Doctorate) or DO (Doctor of Osteopathy)

Education: After medical school, a doctor must attend a post-graduate residency (3-7 years depending on specialty) and pass a series of licensing exams to be licensed to practice medicine in the US.

- Undergraduate (4 years): **Pre-med**
- Medical School (4 years): **Medical student**
- Residency (3-7 years): **Resident**
    - 1st-year resident: **Intern**
    - Less than half their residency training completed: **Junior Resident**
    - More than half their residency training completed: **Senior Resident**
- Optional Fellowship (1-2 years): **Fellow**
- Fully Independent & Board Certified: **Attending**

Specialty: A doctor completes a residency in a single specialty; may specialize further with a fellowship. Specialties include:

- Anesthesiology
- Emergency Medicine
- Dermatology
- Family Medicine
- Internal Medicine
- Obstetrics & Gynecology
- Neurology
- Neurosurgery
- Ophthalmology

- Pathology
- Pediatrics
- Psychiatry
- Radiology
- Surgery

Role:

- Lead multidisciplinary healthcare team.
- Take patient histories and perform a physical exam (H&P).
- Order and interpret labs and imaging.
- Prescribe medications and evaluate response to treatment.
- Perform procedures and surgeries.
- Communicate with patients, family, and other healthcare providers.
- Document care by writing notes.
- Teach medical students and residents (teaching hospitals).
- Inpatient: Admit/discharge patients, 'round' with the team, and manage in-hospital care.
- Outpatient: Manage patients through clinic visits, phone calls, and electronic communications.

Physical Descriptors:

- Long white coat (down to knees) with their name embroidered over breast pocket.
    - Short white coat (ends at waist) indicates student.
- Stethoscope around neck or in pocket of white coat.
- Pager clipped to belt or white coat pocket.
- ID badge.
- Pens in breast pocket.
- Pockets crammed with papers, cell phone, and specialty instruments.
- Medical specialties and outpatient clinics:
    - Business casual clothes.

- Dress shoes.
- Bow ties, tie clip, or no tie/no loose ties.

• Surgical specialties:
- Light blue/light green scrubs from the OR.
- May have hair cover or shoe covers.
- Long hair pulled back; men closely shaved.
- No jewelry, except sometimes a wedding ring on a chain around neck.
- Very clean hands/fingernails, no nail polish.
- Sensible, comfortable footwear, such as tennis shoes or rubber crocs.

• ICU specialties:
- Scrubs from home (embroidered with name) or business casual clothes.
- Sensible shoes.

ROLE

The role of the physician in modern medicine is rapidly changing. Gone are the days of house calls and doctors who would do everything from delivering babies to performing emergency surgeries. Instead, physicians have taken up the mantle of team leader, coordinating a diverse team of healthcare workers to orchestrate care for your character. This changing role means physicians spend less time with their patients and more time writing notes, making phone calls, and conferring with other providers.

A doctor's job is to diagnose and treat patients. They must evaluate your character, figure out what's going wrong, then find a way to fix it. The first step is to collect all the available information, which means performing a history and physical.

> Physical exams almost always include listening to the heart and lungs using a stethoscope.

THE HISTORY AND PHYSICAL

The history and physical, or H&P, is the basic exam all doctors perform; if you've ever had a checkup, you've experienced an H&P. The point of an H&P is for the doctor to better understand why your character is coming to see them. They usually start open-ended– "what brought you in today"–then become more and more focused as the interview progresses. The physical exam is targeted towards the reason your character came in–if your character sprained their ankle, there's no need for the doctor to perform a pelvic exam. In life-threatening situations, the H&P can be extremely narrow, focused only on saving the life.

DIFFERENTIAL DIAGNOSIS

Once the doctor has all the pertinent information, she'll make a list of all the possible diagnoses, called a *differential diagnosis*. A differential diagnosis includes the diagnosis that is most likely to be causing the problem, but it also considers conditions that could be particularly harmful, or even deadly.

TESTING

Once the doctor has a good idea of what's on the differential, she needs to collect objective evidence to support or refute that diagnosis. Sometimes, the evidence from the physical exam is enough. But often, it means ordering and evaluating laboratory tests and medical imaging. Since we already discussed labs and imaging in Ch. 6, I won't go into any more detail here.

TREATMENT

Once the results are back, the doctor develops a treatment plan. This plan could include prescribing a new medication, suggesting a lifestyle change, referring your character to a specialist, or recommending a procedure. Doctors perform lots of procedures, ranging from in-office skin biopsies to complicated surgeries. In the OR, the attending surgeon acts as team leader for the duration of the surgery, though residents may perform the majority of the procedure.

A DAY IN THE LIFE

INPATIENT WARDS

A hospitalist's day starts early, usually by 7 am. First, they sit down and skim their patients' charts. Then comes pass-down, where the night team relays anything important that happened overnight and introduces the team to any new admissions. Afterward, the doctor spends the rest of the morning rounding: checking on patients, adjusting treatment plans, and coordinating care with specialists, therapists, and family members. Throughout the day, doctors accept admissions–patients admitted to the hospital from the emergency department or straight from clinic–and transfers from other wards.

INPATIENT SURGERY:

A surgeon's day typically starts even earlier, often as early as 5 or 6 am. After arriving at the hospital, they receive pass-down from the night team, then check the board to see what surgeries are scheduled for the day. Then, they read through patient charts before very quickly rounding on the floor patients. After rounds, they change into scrubs and head down to the OR, where they will spend most of the day performing surgeries. A surgeon's day is highly unpredictable and varies with their specialty and practice type.

> Surgeon's rounds are notoriously brief–just a few minutes per patient–as they rush to get to the OR.

OUTPATIENT CLINIC:

Clinic doctors include primary care physicians as well as specialists providing outpatient care, such as dermatologists and gynecologists. Their day starts by reviewing the charts of all the patients they're going to see that day and responding to emails and phone messages. Once patients start to arrive–usually around 8 am–they see patient after patient in rapid-fire succession. There's no time for bathroom breaks, never mind actually documenting the visit, so once they've seen all their patients for the day, they spend the next few hours writing notes.

A NOTE ABOUT WHITE COATS

Doctors aren't the only ones to wear white coats anymore. Other medical specialties, such as pharmacists, NPs, and PAs wear them too. No matter their specialty, you can learn a lot about a provider by what is in the pockets of their white coat. Here's what some specialties might carry:

- **Everyone:** Pens, cell phone, scrap paper, water bottle, granola bar, old paperwork they should have thrown in the HIPAA box months ago.
- **Emergency Medicine:** Trauma shears, penlight, miscellaneous wound care supplies.
- **Neurology**: Reflex hammer, penlight, tuning fork
- **Ob/Gyn**: Tape measure
- **Pediatrician**: Toys, otoscope (for looking in ears), tongue depressors
- **Surgery**: Suture removal kit

White coats get heavy; stiff white fabric and full pockets can lead to sore shoulders and tension headaches. If your character wears a white coat, think about what is so important to them that they'll carry it with them everywhere.

BREAKING DOWN THE CLICHÉS: DOCTOR STEREOTYPES

There are too many doctor tropes to include them all in this chapter. I'll start with one that is, unfortunately, pretty accurate.

THE REAL DOCTOR

"Excuse me, when am I going to see the doctor?"

"I am your doctor."

"No. The real doctor."

Less of a trope and more of an unfortunate reality, young, female, and POC physicians–especially those who are any combination of the three–are mistaken for nurses (or janitors!) on an almost daily basis. This misbranding can be subtle- asking female physicians for nursing-level care–to blatantly refusing to call a female physician "doctor." Every female physician I know has had patients who insisted on calling them "nurse," even after they've introduced themselves as the doctor, or who refuse to acknowledge the treatment plan until it comes from a man's mouth. If a patient has a male nurse, they may direct all their questions to him, putting the poor man in the awkward situation of either answering the question–not only insulting the doctor but risking providing the wrong answer–or repeatedly trying to redirect the patient and undermining the nurse-patient relationship.

This type of bias is bad for everyone. Not only does it undermine the hard work and achievements of female and POC physicians, but it is straight-up dangerous. Nurses have different skills and training than doctors–expecting a doctor to provide nursing-level care is just as dangerous as expecting a nurse to provide physician-level care.

And while, in the real world, the dismissal of female, young, and POC physicians is disheartening and frustrating, in writing, it presents some intriguing opportunities. Character-building, interpersonal tension, moral quandaries; it's all there, should you choose to use it.

DR. BADBOY

"You can't do that! It's against protocol."

"Screw protocol! I'm here to save lives, not read textbooks!"

Medicine is an art, yes, but it is first and foremost a science. Doctors don't just pull treatments and procedures out of thin air; they make recommendations based on scientific evidence. And that scientific evidence is always changing. To keep up with the ever-changing face of medicine, doctors are expected to read medical journals and incorporate those findings into their medical practice. At academic teaching hospitals, this mentality means daily lunchtime presentations, weekly journal clubs, and monthly Grand Rounds. Medical students and residents are expected to memorize seminal studies and regurgitate the findings on command. Most physicians would have way more respect for someone who can cite the latest findings on alpha-synuclein levels in the diagnosis of Parkinson's disease, than for someone who immediately jumps to the diagnosis without bothering with pesky tests.

Also, Dr. Badboy is going to get his a$$ sued. A 2017 study found that over 55% of physicians have been sued in their lifetime, and that number only gets higher for procedural specialties, with 85% of surgeons and Ob/Gyn having been sued at some point in their career.[1] To successfully defend against malpractice, physicians go out of their way to document every move they make, whether that's prescribing medications, performing a procedure, or simply providing medical advice. In that documentation, they not only describe what was done but why–and 'because it sounded like a good idea at the time' won't cut it. Without scientific evidence on his side, Dr. Badboy is going to have a hard time.

DOCTOR STEREOTYPES BY SPECIALTY

I recognize that I just wrote a whole section on *avoiding* stereotyping doctors. But sometimes, stereotypes exist for a reason. And who better to stereotype doctors than other doctors? So, here's a list of stereotypes by specialty.

Anesthesiologist: Lazy (take naps during surgery); enjoy getting high on their own meds.

Cardiothoracic Surgeon: Cadillac of doctors. Hard-working. Lifesaving. Super rich. Full of themselves.

Cardiologist: Medical doctor with a surgeon's attitude. Hardcore. Fat phobic.

Dermatology: Rich and privileged. Never miss their afternoon tee time.

Emergency Dr.: Cowboys, thrill-seekers, adrenaline junkies. The worst doctors in the hospital.

Family Medicine: Barely passed medical school. Idealists.

Gastroenterologist: Poop doctor. Wealthy. Laidback lifestyle.

General Surgeons: Arrogant, abrasive, mean. Hates talking to patients. Terrible bedside manner.

Internal Medicine (Hospitalist): Default doctor. Long-winded. Overly academic. Boring. Spends all day rounding.

Ob/Gyn: Male = Gay. Female = Overworked goddess, Catty, or Butch B*tch.

Orthopedic Surgeons: Jocks; male-centric egoists.

Neurologist: Armchair doctors, nerds in bowties. Can't help their patients.

Nephrology: Proof you can be the nerd amongst nerds. Dialysis doctors.

Neurosurgeon: Workaholics. A special kind of crazy (remember that 7-year residency?).

Pathologist: No people skills. Off-center, off-putting personality. Only works with dead people.

Pediatrics: Mr. Rogers in a white coat.

Psychiatry: Fake doctors, daddy issues.

Radiology: Vampires who spend all day in the dark. Poor people skills.

Remember, these are stereotypes. Knowing the stereotype means you can not only avoid falling into them but actively subvert them.

9. NURSES

Education:

- Licensed Practical Nurse (LPN).
  - 1-Year accreditation does not require an undergraduate degree.

- Registered Nurse (RN).
  - Most nurses are RNs.
  - Requires an undergraduate degree in nursing.
    - Bachelor of Science in Nursing (BSN).
    - Associate Degree in Nursing (AND).

- Advanced Practice Nurse.
  - NP, CRNA, CNS, CNM.
  - DNP.

- Ph.D. in Nursing.

Role:

- Evaluate and monitor patient condition and response to treatment.
- Monitor vital signs.
- Communicate with patients, family, and healthcare team.
- Patient advocate.
- Administer and evaluate response to medications.
- Document care provided.
- Assist with surgeries and procedures.
- Wound care.
- Double-check physician orders.

Physical Descriptors:

- Brightly colored, loose-fitting scrubs.
    - Surgical nurses wear OR scrubs, scrub caps, and shoe covers.
- Comfortable shoes.
- Stethoscope around neck.
- ID badge.
- Pockets filled with supplies.

ROLE:

The role of nurses is much broader than many people think. Nurses can be found in pretty much every subsection of healthcare, from the ICU and Operating Room to clinics, schools, and home health. Many nurses practice independently or as part of a physician-led team.

Nurses are the first line of healthcare and often have significantly more patient interaction than their physician counterparts. The vital role of nursing, in both inpatient and outpatient, cannot be underestimated. Like physicians, nurses have a wide variety of roles, ranging from independent outpatient practice to surgical assists.

A DAY IN THE LIFE:

Inpatient: Most inpatient nurses work either 8- or 12-hour shifts.[1] The day starts with a morning huddle and pass-down from the night team. Then, the nurse will begin his morning rounds, passing out medications, checking blood sugar, and assisting with daily activities, such as eating or toileting. Whenever he gets the chance, he'll catch up on charting. In the afternoon, he'll repeat those rounds, introducing himself to any new patients. He'll also make sure to carve out time to communicate important changes to both the physician team and the patient and their family. At the end of his shift, he'll make sure everything is properly documented and will hand off his patients to the night team.

Emergency: An ED nurse's day is highly variable. Like inpatient RNs, ED nurses usually work 12-hour shifts, but that's where the resemblance stops. ED nurses don't have a consistent set of patients–instead, they'll be assigned patients based on the medical complexity determined by the triage nurse. Depending on who walks through the door, they could be doing anything from checking blood pressures to picking maggots out of a necrotic wound.[2]

Surgery: Surgical nurses provide a wide variety of patient care, from providing pre- and post-operative care to assisting in surgery. An OR nurse will begin her day by checking in with the surgeon and the perioperative clinical coordinator to find out what surgeries are on the schedule.

There are several different roles for surgical nurses. A **scrub nurse** scrubs in before anyone else, prepares and counts the surgical tools, and hands the surgeon the proper tools. A **surgical first assist** assists the surgeon during the procedure. A **circulating nurse's** job is to make sure the flow of surgery goes well by performing safety checks, helping the surgeon and her assistants gown in, and taking notes as the surgery progresses.

> "Gowning in" is the process by which surgeons and assistants dress in sterilized blue gowns to prepare for surgery.

Home Health: A home health nurse practices independently, traveling to patients' homes to provide medical care. Care provided can range from hospice care to home safety analysis.

BREAKING DOWN THE CLICHÉS:

You might not be surprised to find there are a lot of stereotypes and clichés surrounding nursing.

THE HANDMAIDEN

"Yes, Doctor."

Every Fictional Nurse

The trope of the subservient, brainless, and pretty nurse who exists only to meekly follow the handsome doctor's orders is as pervasive as it is damaging. Nurses are intelligent, independent practitioners with their own autonomy, education, and unique skill set. They are the front line of patient care, interacting one-on-one with patients and family. While doctors (generally) write the orders, nurses are the ones who carry them out. If a nurse disagrees, doesn't understand, or is uncomfortable with those orders, it is a critical part of their job to confront the physician and ask for clarification. Lives are saved through this system of mutual trust and respect.

NAUGHTY NURSE:

Nurse walks in wearing a tight white outfit

Bends over

Puts boobs in male protagonist's face *Jiggles them around while fixing his BP cuff*

In the 'Naughty Nurse' trope, a character (usually male) hypersexualizes his female nurse. Or the nurse delights in the sexual attention from her patients. Either way, she's turning hospital beds into tents.

The trope of the naughty nurse is so overused that it can be found as the titular character in romance novels, pornography, and Halloween costumes. But female nurses, like most professional women, are more concerned with doing their job than with turning on their patients.

A nurse's job is far from sexy. From monitoring bowel movements to changing crusty wound dressings, nurses—not doctors—are the ones who deal with some of the most disgusting aspects of medicine on a daily basis. This reality quickly leads to a no-nonsense attitude, as well as a pragmatic approach to attire. Scrubs tend to be loose, rather than skintight, and many nurses (though certainly not all) are much too busy to bother with things like wearing makeup or doing their hair. Why bother getting dressed up when you're going to end up smelling like a *C. Diff* infection?

> **Clostridium dificile**, affectionately known as "C. diff" has a unique smell so pungent, providers joke they can diagnose it from the hallway.

But this no-nonsense attitude doesn't stop patients from sexualizing their nurses, and many of them act on those impulses. A 2020 study found that over 43% of female nurses had experienced sexual harassment.[3] Nearly 75% of the time, the perpetrator was a patient or the patient's family.[3] The remaining 25% were coworkers.[3]

ANGEL NURSE:

A Nurse Will Always Give Us Hope, an Angel with a Stethoscope.

While I appreciate the gratitude patients feel towards their nurses, stereotyping nurses as angels sets an impossible standard. If nurses are angels, they won't mind working grueling shifts for too-little pay or batting away the attentions of patients (or coworkers) fixated on the naughty-nurse stereotype. They won't get irritable after a sixteen-hour shift,

> A **census** is the number of patients the provider is responsible for caring for.

and they certainly won't make any mistakes despite having an overloaded census. If nurses are angels, then they won't have all the fun, human range of emotions that makes for good writing.

B*TCH NURSE:

"You didn't say please."

**Indistinguishable wheezing*

"You won't get your inhaler until I hear you say 'please.'"

Ah, misogyny at its finest. If a nurse stands up for herself or is high up in the chain of command and must make some tough choices, then she's not an angel anymore–she's reached the level of b*tch nurse. Epitomized by Nurse Ratched from *One Flew Over the Cuckoo's Nest,* a b*tch nurse is cruel, sadistic, in-control, and, worst of all, unfeminine.

MURSE

"What do you do for a living?"

"I'm a nurse."

**Nervous laughter* "Come on bro, what do you really do?"*

"I'm a nurse."

Male nurses tend to be portrayed in one of two ways; they are either bulky and intimidating–more of a bouncer than a nurse–or they are less of a man. Nursing is still considered a feminine profession and men who choose it are unfairly subjected to scrutiny. Did they only go into nursing because they couldn't get into medical school? Are they somehow lazy or less qualified? Do they just want to get into their fellow nurse's pants?

And then, there's the whole dating thing. Male doctors dating female nurses? Sexy. Female doctors dating male nurses? Sleazy.

The idea that male nurses are anything less than perfectly normal is ridiculous. Nurses come in all shapes, sizes, colors, and genders. Your writing should reflect this reality.

10. ADVANCED PRACTICE PROVIDERS (APPS)

Education:

Physician Assistant: Master's Degree

Advanced Nurse Practitioner: Master of Science in Nursing (MSN) or Doctoral Nursing Program (DNP)

Credentials:

Physician Assistant: PA-C

Advanced Practice Nurse:

- Nurse Practitioner (NP or DNP)
- Clinical Nurse Specialist (CNS)

Certified Registered Nurse Anesthetist (CRNA)

- Certified Nurse Midwife (CNM)

Role (PA, NP):

- Take a patient history and perform a physical exam (H&P).
- Order and interpret labs and imaging.
- Prescribe medications and evaluate response to treatment.
- Communicate with patients, family, and other healthcare providers.
- Document care by writing notes.
- Inpatient: Work on an interdisciplinary team and manage in-hospital care.
- Outpatient: Manage patients through clinic visits, phone calls, and electronic communications.

> Look familiar? The role and description of Advanced Practitioners are almost identical to those of physicians. The main differences are that APNs do not perform complex surgical procedures and are rarely the leaders of the healthcare team.

Specialty Roles:
- CNM: Provides women's healthcare, including labor and delivery.
- CNS: Specializes in population health, research, and nursing education.
- CRNA: Administers anesthesia and monitors patients throughout procedures.[1]

Physical Descriptors:
- Long white coat with their name embroidered over breast pocket.
- Stethoscope, Pager, and ID badge.
- Pockets crammed with papers, cell phone, and specialty instruments.
- Medical specialties (or surgical Clinic):
    o Business casual clothes, dress shoes, no loose ties.
- Surgical specialties:
    o Light blue/light green scrubs, hair and shoe covers, comfortable shoes.
    o Hair pulled back, men closely shaved, clean hands, no jewelry.

Advanced Practitioners are healthcare providers that provide care at a level similar to that of physicians, though they did not go to medical school. Advanced Practitioners can diagnose and treat patients, prescribe medications, order diagnostic tests, and make important medical decisions. As the US healthcare system attempts to cut costs and administer healthcare to an aging population, APPs make up more and more of the healthcare workforce. If your character goes for a checkup, they'll probably be seen by an APP rather than a doctor. Advanced practitioners come in two flavors: Physician Assistants (PAs) and Advanced Nurse Practitioners (APNs).

PHYSICIAN ASSISTANT (PA)

The title "Physician Assistant" is pretty misleading–PAs are so much more than assistants! In the clinic, they diagnose and treat patients independently. In hospitals, they work on multidisciplinary healthcare teams, managing floor patients, taking admissions, and preparing discharges. If they're in a surgical specialty, PAs might manage the post-operative floor patients while the doctor is in surgery, or they may act as First Assist in the OR.

PAs can be found in any specialty in the hospital, from primary care to cardiothoracic surgery. Unlike doctors, PAs don't undergo residency and instead receive much of their specialized training on the job.[2] This lack of specialization means that a PA can jump easily jump between specialties. That isn't to say that PAs aren't well trained–their two-year Master's degree is brutal and highly focused on early mastery of clinical skills. But the lack of a required residency gives PAs an incredible amount of career flexibility. Whenever a kid asks my advice on what they want to be when they grow up, I tell them don't go to medical school, become a PA instead.

ADVANCE PRACTICE NURSES (APNS)

Unlike PAs, DOs, and MDs, most APNs decide to become advanced practitioners only after they've worked as an RN for a few years. And unlike PAs, APNs tend to specialize based on the certification program they pursue. There are several different types of APNs.

NURSE PRACTITIONERS

Most Nurse Practitioners have doctoral-level degrees (DNPs). Their scope of practice is determined by the area of their study. NPs can work on inpatient specialty teams, like cardiology or neurosurgery, in a specialty private practice, or they can work independently as a primary care provider. They can prescribe Schedule II drugs, such as Morphine and Adderall.

CLINICAL NURSE SPECIALIST

Clinical Nurse Specialists, who can have Master or Doctoral level training, focus on systems-level nursing. They are often seen in hospitals, schools, and community health clinics, applying evidence-based research. They are educators, researchers, and consultants who focus more on population-level care than individual clinical care.[3]

> Schedule II Drugs are the highest level of legal controlled substances.

CERTIFIED REGISTERED NURSE ANESTHETIST (CRNA)

A CRNA is the nurse equivalent of an anesthesiologist. They interview and examine potential recipients of anesthesia, intubate and extubate, administer the anesthesia, and monitor the patient during the procedure and recovery. Technically, they do all this under the supervision of an MD anesthesiologist, but in practice, they function quite independently. In fact, in rural hospitals, a CRNA may be the only person in the hospital with the ability to administer anesthesia.[2]

CERTIFIED NURSE MIDWIFE (CNM)

A CNM provides women's healthcare, ranging from routine Pap smears to delivering babies. They can prescribe birth control pills, give vaccinations, and treat sexually transmitted infections (STIs). CNMs can provide obstetric care throughout pregnancy and can facilitate births at home, at birthing facilities, or even in the hospital.

CNMs mostly provide care to women with uncomplicated pregnancies–if anything goes wrong, care may need to be transferred to an Obstetrics/Gynecology doctor.

INTER-PROVIDER RELATIONS

As the need for providers increases, and hospitals attempt to cut costs, the US healthcare system is increasingly relying on Advanced Practitioners to provide physician-level care. This shift is a source of friction between doctors and their non-physician counterparts. Many doctors believe APPs do not have sufficient training to practice independently; APPs point to a lack of evidence for this claim. And while the details of this argument are too nuanced to go into here, note that this friction is a potential source of tension between characters. How would your character feel if they went to a doctor's appointment, and in turn were seen by a PA? If your character is pregnant, would she choose to be seen by a midwife or an Ob/Gyn doctor? Would your character treat an NP with less respect, believing that she is "just a nurse," despite her doctoral-level training? If your character needs surgery, would they be comfortable knowing that a nurse is performing the anesthesia?

BREAKING DOWN THE CLICHÉ: THE PHYSICIAN'S ASSISTANT

"Doctor, we need to figure out your schedule for the next month."

Waves hand irritably "Contact my PA. She'll deal with the details."

Whoever named "Physician Assistants" did a terrible job. PAs are not assistants in the traditional sense of the word. They don't take phone calls, coordinate schedules, or write the doctor's notes for them; they're independent practitioners who work under the umbrella of a leading physician. PAs see patients independently, prescribe medications, order tests, and write their own d*mn notes. The only time PAs assist with anything is during surgery.

> Take out that possessive "'s"! PA don't belong to the doctor they work with.

The same is true of other Advanced Practitioners–they work *with* physicians, not under them. APPs have their own licensing and certification, their own education, and their own practice. And while some things require physician 'supervision'–for instance, a doctor's name will appear on a prescription alongside the PA's name–that supervision is often quite limited.

So, if APPs can do all the same things as doctors, why do we have doctors?

Good question. Doctors are more highly specialized, and they can perform procedures that APPs can't. They have a broad education with an emphasis on a deep understanding of the human body at its most fundamental level and years of required training in their chosen specialty before they can practice independently. But what's the difference, functionally, between a primary care doctor and a primary care APP?

Depends on who you ask. Like I said earlier, the expanding scope of practice of APPs is a source of friction for many. And I'll leave it at that.

11. EMERGENCY MEDICAL SERVICE (EMS) PROVIDERS

Types

- Emergency Medical Responder (First Responder)
- Emergency Medical Technician (EMT)
- Paramedic

Education: High school diploma plus…

- EMT-basic (EMT-b): 3-month course + state certification
- Paramedic: EMT-b + 2-year paramedic training course

Role

- Respond to 911 calls
- Provide medical support and stabilization
- Triage multiple patients
- Transport patients to the emergency department
- Transport medically fragile patients between medical facilities (EMT-b)
- Provide Basic Life Support (EMT-b) or Advanced Cardiac Life Support (Paramedic)
- Intubate and manually ventilate, read EKGs, administer certain medications (Paramedic)
- Communicate with law enforcement, patients and family, and hospital staff
- Document care given

Identification

- Uniform: Collared shirt (blue, black, or white) with cargo pants
- Patch with the logo of ambulance company on shoulder or above breast pocket
    o May have an additional patch with Star of Life
- ID badge

- Belt with pager
- Pens in breast pocket
- Pants pockets filled with supplies, including trauma shears and bandages
- All-weather gear (jackets, reflective vests) with ambulance company logo

EMS providers are so much more than ambulance drivers. Along with firefighters and police, they're the first to the scene of an emergency and the first to provide medical care. The medical care provided can range anywhere from a Band-Aid to intubation, and everything in between.

There are three types of EMS providers: Emergency Medical Responders (EMRs), Emergency Medical Technicians (EMTs), and Paramedics.

EMERGENCY MEDICAL RESPONDERS

Emergency Medical Responders, also known as First Responders, are the first ones to arrive at the scene of an emergency. Usually, they're firefighters or police. The job of a First Responder is to keep your character from dying until the ambulance arrives. They know CPR and how to open an airway, how to protect C-spine, can slap a bandage on a hemorrhaging wound, perform the Heimlich, give Naloxone, and maybe stabilize a broken limb. But that's about it. An EMR training course takes about 8 hours. First Responders have significant training in other areas, but their medical training is relatively limited. Once EMS shows up, it's the Responder's job to follow commands and ensure the EMTs are working in a safe environment.

> Protecting C-Spine is vital to preventing your character from severing their spinal cord (Ch. 12)

EMERGENCY MEDICAL TECHNICIAN (EMT)

An EMT is an EMS provider capable of providing basic life support, such as CPR and airway maintenance, along with several other noninvasive– but potentially lifesaving– techniques. For instance, EMTs are trained to recognize the signs of low blood sugar, take a patient's blood sugar, and administer glucose. They can also take vital signs, give oxygen, ventilate using a BMV, control hemorrhage (including tie a tourniquet), maintain an airway, place airway devices, stabilize C-spine, splint an injured limb, even deliver babies and provide newborn resuscitation.

> Actually driving the ambulance is not a part of EMT training; EMTs get to learn that on the job!

EMTs have a limited number of medications they are allowed to administer. While the exact rules vary by state, some examples include:[1]

- Activated charcoal — for ingested toxins
- Albuterol — for asthma or other breathing emergencies
- Aspirin — for heart attacks
- Epinephrine (via EpiPen or vial) — for anaphylaxis
- Nitroglycerin — for heart attacks
- Oral Glucose — for low blood sugar
- Oxygen — any emergency where your character's breathing or heart is compromised.
- Tylenol — for fever and pain control

> There are very few conditions that oxygen can make worse. If your character is sick, the EMTs will probably slap on an oxygen mask, even if they aren't overtly having trouble breathing.

However, to administer these medications, EMTs need permission from Medical Command. The exceptions are for lifesaving drugs–aspirin, epinephrine, oral glucose, and oxygen–which can be administered immediately and permission from Command acquired retrospectively.

EMT-PARAMEDIC (PARAMEDIC)

Becoming a paramedic is a commitment. Though each state has different licensing requirements, paramedics must first be EMTs, and must have at least 6 months of on-the-job experience–most have more. The paramedic training course then takes up to two years, requiring between 1,200-1,800 hours to complete.[3] Many paramedics complete the training while working as an EMT.

Once their training and certification are complete, paramedics have a host of skills. They are trained in Advanced Cardiac Life Support, meaning they can intubate, read EKGs, and administer cardiac medications These include:[2]

> An ambulance isn't a bus–it's a rig!

- Rapid Sequence Intubation, including paralyzing medications
- IV insertion and maintenance
- Giving IV fluids and medications
- Breathing treatments, such as Albuterol
- Giving cardiac medications, such as Amiodarone or Atropine
- Giving psychiatric medications, such as Haldol or Ativan

A DAY IN THE LIFE

EMTs and paramedics work on ambulances, usually in twelve-hour shifts. They work in pairs; often an EMT is paired with a paramedic. When a call comes in from the medical dispatcher, the team drives out to the call, both sitting up front. The dispatcher tells the team about the call and determines whether they'll need to use lights and sirens. Once they arrive, one team member (usually the paramedic) will grab the jump bag–a portable bag carrying basic medical supplies–and walk over to the patient while the other gets the gurney out of the back. Depending on the call, the paramedic may also grab other important equipment, like their medication bag or the EKG machine. Then, they'll talk to the patient, working quickly to figure out what is wrong and which treatments, if any, they need to provide. If your character needs to be taken to the hospital, they'll put them on the stretcher and load them into the back of the ambulance.

> Not all ambulance calls end up in trips to the hospital.

On the drive to the Emergency Department, the team determines whether lights and sirens are needed based on the severity of your character's affliction. Usually, the EMT drives while the paramedic stays in back with the patient. Oh, and no, it's not actually legal for ambulances to speed. Even with lights and sirens, they are still technically supposed to follow the speed limit.

> There may be significant down time between calls, or they might be running nonstop. This can change day-to-day, location-to-location.

BREAKING DOWN THE CLICHÉ: WE CHEAT DEATH

> *"Wow, today was really amazing."*
>
> *"Yeah. Look at all those lives we saved!"*

Yes, EMS personnel can save lives. Sometimes. If they're lucky, and they get to the right patient at exactly the right time. It just isn't the norm.

Most calls are pretty mundane. EMS personnel provide transfers to SNFs, rides to dialysis, or transport comatose patients to their annual physical. Many calls to 911 are pretty inane: "my son fell off his bicycle," "I slammed my finger in a car door," or "I haven't pooped in four days." There are calls for behavioral emergencies– usually because the police aren't equipped to deal with psychiatric patients–and calls for garden-variety aches and pains. And then, there are the patients they can't save: the helmet-less motorcyclist who hit a tree, the car that plunged 100 feet down a ravine, the teenage boy who blew his brains out with his father's hunting rifle.

There's a reason EMTs and paramedics are notorious for their jaded attitudes. Like ED nurses and doctors, EMS personnel have to deal with the strangest mix of human stupidity, selfishness, and sorrow. It's enough to make anyone crazy. Those who succeed in these fields find a way to celebrate the few victories they're given. Those who don't burn out.

12. OTHER HEALTHCARE PERSONNEL

MEDICINE IS COMPRISED OF so much more than just doctors and nurses. The buzzword in medicine right now is the "multidisciplinary team." And nowhere is this multidisciplinary team more apparent than in the hospital. This section will give a brief introduction to several other healthcare professionals. I certainly don't expect you to write every single one into your story. Instead, think about each of these professions and how they relate to the healthcare professional in your story. Are you having a physician character do the job of a social worker? A nurse doing the job of a CNA? I understand wanting to streamline your characters—you don't want to have to introduce five characters when one could do—but make sure that one character is in the right profession.

COUNSELOR

Role: Provide support and guidance for those dealing with mental illness, grief, substance abuse, marital strife, or other life stressors.

Degree: Licensed Professional Counselor (LPC) or Master of Social Work in counseling (MSW).

Settings: Hospital, Psychiatric Ward, Intensive Outpatient facilities, private clinics, schools.

A counselor will work with your character to provide guidance and strategies for overcoming personal challenges. Counselors tend to specialize; a marriage counselor will work with couples, while a substance use counselor will work with those struggling with addiction. Though they certainly can provide one-on-one therapy, they can also lead group therapy and professional education projects. In the hospital, counselors are usually found in the psychiatric ward, where they lead group therapy and provide individual counseling for admitted patients. However, those are not the only counselors in the hospital. Grief counselors help families come to terms with a recent loss. Child

> Though the terms are sometimes used interchangeably, counselors are not psychologists or psychiatrists.

life counselors help children deal with the stress of a hospital admission or having a sick parent. In the ED, crisis counselors provide victims of suicide attempts, sexual assault, natural disasters, and domestic violence with psychological first aid to help your character cope with their recent crisis.

NURSE'S AIDE (CNA)

Role: Assist nurses with daily patient care.

Credentials: Certified Nursing Assistant (CNA).

Settings: Hospitals, Rehabilitation Hospitals, Nursing Facilities & Skilled Nursing Facilities (SNF), Long-term Care Facilities, Adult Daycare Centers.

Identifiers: Brightly colored or patterned scrubs, stethoscope, and comfortable shoes. May be difficult to differentiate from nurses without looking at their name badge.

CNAs assist nurses and help patients with their activities of daily living (ADLs), assisting with bathing, feeding, dressing, turning, and toileting. They can take vital signs and answer call lights. If your character is hospitalized, they're almost guaranteed to have a CNA helping to take care of them.

OCCUPATIONAL THERAPIST (OT)

Role: Help patients perform their daily tasks after accident or illness.

Credentials: Master or Doctorate in Occupational Therapy (MTD/DTD).

Settings: Hospitals, clinics, nursing homes, private homes.

Identifiers: Business-casual clothes or scrubs. No stethoscope but may carry a bag full of assistive devices plus their laptop.

An occupational therapist's job is to help a patient complete their activities of daily living (ADLs). Whether it's helping someone who's had a stroke relearn how to hold a spoon or teaching a new amputee how to use the toilet on their own, OTs are essential for helping your character get back on their feet. OTs will also help your character learn to use assistive technology (like wheelchairs or language boards) and will educate their caregivers in the best ways to help your character return to their life.

PATIENT SITTER

Role: Monitor people who might be a danger to themselves or others.

Credentials: On-the-job Training.

Locations: Hospital patient rooms, particularly in the ED.

If your character is suicidal, demented, delirious, or otherwise not in their right state of mind, they may need a patient sitter in the room with them 24-7 to monitor them and make sure they don't hurt themselves. The sitter doesn't provide any medical care, but they can keep your character from trying to stand on their broken leg or pulling out their IV. Many CNAs also work as sitters, providing both personal care (changing, bathing, feeding) and close monitoring.

PATIENT TRANSPORT

Role: Transport patients around the hospital.

Credentials: On-the-job training.

Settings: Hospital, Clinics (rarely).

Identifiers: Hospital-supplied scrubs (usually a different color from the OR scrubs) and comfortable shoes. May wear shoe covers and scrub caps if transporting to the OR.

Contrary to popular media, doctors and nurses don't spend their time wheeling patients around the hospital. That's the job of hospital transport—people trained to safely assist your character in and out of wheelchairs, navigate crowded hallways, transport the deceased to the morgue, and even ferry medical samples to and from the lab.

PHARMACIST

Role: Fill prescriptions and counsel patients on the appropriate use of their medication.

Education: Doctorate in Pharmacy (PharmD).

Locations: Pharmacies–Hospital, Commercial, or Compounding.

Identifiers: Long white coat over business-casual clothes.

Pharmacists do a lot more than just fill prescriptions and count pills. In fact, pharmacists don't count out the pills themselves–they have pharmacy technicians who do that. Instead, the pharmacist's role centers around patient safety and education. If an idiot doctor* tries to order an antibiotic for a patient who is allergic to said antibiotic, they call that doctor up and calmly walk them through how to properly choose which antibiotic to prescribe. Pharmacists monitor drug therapy, screen for contraindications like allergies, pregnancy, and drug-drug interactions. They can even administer vaccinations and some medications.

> *Like me

PHYSICAL THERAPIST (PT)

Role: Improve quality of life through movement and exercise.

Education: Doctor of Physical Therapy (DPT).

Settings: Hospitals, clinics, nursing homes, even private homes.

Identifiers: Scrubs or stretchy business casual clothes they can move in–think fancy yoga pants–and running shoes. Carries a bag with PT supplies and laptop.

Equipment: Resistance bands, weights and dumbbells, exercise mats, tens machine, exercise ball, workout equipment (treadmill, stationary bike, elliptical, rowing machine).

Physical therapists use exercise to treat a manage a wide variety of ailments. Whether it's carpal tunnel, low back pain, stroke, arthritis, joint replacement, spine injury, or horrific burns, physical therapists will have an exercise for that. In fact, after being discharged from the hospital, many patients–especially victims of stroke, amputation, and severe burns or wounds–will spend anywhere from a few days to several weeks at a rehabilitation hospital before going home.[1]

> See Ch. 7 for more on rehab hospitals.

RESPIRATORY THERAPIST

Role: Care for people with trouble breathing. Administer breathing treatments and pulmonary function testing.

Degree: Certified Respiratory Therapist (CRT) or Registered Respiratory Therapist (RRT).

> Most practicing respiratory therapists have the more advanced RRT credentials.

Settings: Hospitals, pulmonary clinics, sleep clinics, private homes.

Identifiers: Scrubs, stethoscope, bag full of assistive devices such as nebulizers and BiPAP/CPAP machines.

Respiratory therapists are often seen in ICUs, wards, and EDs, administering oxygen and breathing treatments, managing ventilators, and measuring lung function.

SPEECH & LANGUAGE PATHOLOGIST (SLP)

Role: Help patients speak, swallow, and communicate.

Degree: Master's in Speech-Language Pathology (MSLP).

Settings: Hospitals, clinics, nursing homes, private homes.

Identifiers: Business-casual clothes or scrubs. No stethoscope but will carry a bag full of assistive devices plus their laptop.

In a hospital or rehab clinic, SLPs perform the critical function of evaluating a patient's swallow, then providing therapy to help them improve. Swallowing is–unsurprisingly–an incredibly important aspect of recovery. If your character has a stroke, make sure they have an SLP evaluate their swallow–unless, of course, you're looking for an excuse for your character to choke or aspirate.

But SLPs do so much more than swallow evals. They help children overcome lisps and stutters, teach stroke victims how to talk again, and help nonverbal people learn to communicate despite their barriers. They can work with a wide range of characters, ranging from children on the autism spectrum to victims of stroke or traumatic brain injury.

> Aspiration pneumonia occurs when your character is breathing in their food, called aspirating, instead of swallowing it.

SOCIAL WORKER:

Education: Bachelor of Social Work (BSW) or Master's in Social Work (LCSW).

Role: Help patients navigate the complex healthcare system and advocate for them.

Settings: Hospitals, Rehabilitation facilities, Community.

Identifiers: Business-casual clothes, sturdy shoes.

Good social workers are worth their weight in gold. Without one, the doctor will end up spending hours

> Social workers can also provide counseling.

on the phone fighting with insurance companies, government programs, and stepdown facilities. Social workers also provide critical advocacy for your marginalized characters, particularly those who are homeless, struggling with addiction, or disabled.[2] A social worker can keep your character from falling through the cracks. Duties of social workers include:[3]

- Assessing patient social, financial, and environmental needs
- Helping patients navigate the health care system
- Guiding patients and families through grief or trauma
- Providing extra support to children, veterans, and those with disabilities
- Educating hospital staff
- Discharging planning
- Evaluating signs of abuse, neglect, and/or trauma

A social worker could be the unsung hero of your story. Who finds your character a spot in the state-supported rehabilitation hospital when they have nowhere else to go? Who connects them to a shelter so that they aren't discharged to the street? Who finds a psychiatrist willing to take your character on? You guessed it. Social workers are the answer to many of healthcare's stickiest problems—and they might just be the realistic solution your story needs.

> Discharge planning–figuring out where your character will go after their hospitalization–is hugely important and complex. Without it, your character is at high risk of readmission and adverse events. They could even end up being on the street!

BREAKING DOWN THE CLICHÉ: SUPER-DOC

Dr. Bigheart greets your character as they arrive at the ED, taking their history from the paramedic as they race to the OR. The anesthetist is running late, so Dr. Bigheart goes ahead and starts the anesthesia himself before performing the surgery. When your character wakes, Dr. Bigheart is sitting at their bedside, praying. He offers them an extra pillow and some ice chips and, when he realizes your character hasn't urinated in twelve hours, straight caths them himself. As he speaks with your character, Dr. Bigheart notices something off about them, and carefully begins to question them about the accident. When your character admits, tearfully, that the accident was a suicide attempt, Dr. Bigheart holds their hand while they cry, prescribes an antidepressant, then offers to stay with them until they feel better.

No one person can do all of this. Never mind that doctors are simply too busy to provide this level of continuity of care; they also lack the necessary training. Doctors are neither superheroes nor are they magically skilled in all things healthcare. An anesthesiologist has a very different skill set from an emergency room doctor. Even a cardiothoracic surgeon's skills and knowledge base are vastly different from that of an orthopedic surgeon. Physicians specialize, and for good reason; the depth of knowledge required is simply too great to focus on more than one or two aspects of medicine.

The other unrealistic aspect of the trope of the super-doc is how much time they spend with the patient. TV shows often show entire teams of doctors spending hours trying to figure out the treatment plan for a single patient, or personally accompanying the patient to their procedures and imaging studies. To quote my favorite meme, "Ain't nobody got time for that."[4] Doctors have a high census, caring for an average of twenty patients per day.[5] On average, doctors see each patient for nine minutes and spend only 18% of their time in direct patient care.[5]

PART 3: MEDICINE BASICS

13. APPROACH TO AN EMERGENCY

Your protagonist—let's call him Al—is driving home from a CPR class with his wife, Aida, on a dark country road. Tired and cranky after spending his Saturday on a class he's sure he's never going to use, Al stews in silence. A motorcyclist comes roaring up behind them, then passes, despite the double-yellow line. Al flips him the bird—the idiot isn't even wearing a helmet. Suddenly, headlights appear around the bend. The motorcyclist swerves in front of Al's car, narrowly avoiding a head-on collision. Al slams of the brakes, but the motorcyclist hits a pothole and careens out of control. Aida screams as the motorcyclist is catapulted off his bike and into a ditch.

Al pulls over to the curb and they both jump out. They find the driver lying on his back a few feet away, his jeans and t-shirt ripped and bloody.

WHEW, THERE'S A LOT TO unpack there. If you're writing a story about a medical emergency, it's important to know how the pros handle it. Even if your character isn't a pro, they should follow these general steps—unless you want them to look like an idiot.

Al races to the motorcyclist's side, kneeling beside him. He calls for the man and shakes his shoulder, but he doesn't respond. So, Al performs a sternal rub—a technique he learned just that morning—raking his knuckles over the man's breastbone. The man moans but makes no other response. Meanwhile, Aida gets out her cellphone and calls 911.

> A sternal rub is a painful stimulus used to help determine a character's level of consciousness. Try it on your friend or partner next time they fall asleep in front of the TV, and you'll see how effective it can be.

The first step is always to call 911. There might be some situations where your character can't (or won't), but if that's the case, you're going to need a d*mn good reason why.

While your character is waiting for the ambulance to arrive, they'll care for the victim by following the ABCs.

THE C-ABCS

In an emergency, medical professionals prioritize the stabilization of the ABCs—Airway, Breathing, and Circulation—and in that order. If your character has any medical training (or common sense), they will too. After all, you can't live long without oxygen. Let's go through the c-ABCs as your character might if they came upon someone having an emergency.

CPR

The little case "c" in the c-ABCs stands for CPR. If your character sees someone drop, the very first step is to check for a pulse. If they don't have one, proceed straight to CPR (Ch.15). If they do have a pulse, move on to the next step: airway.

AIRWAY WITH C-SPINE PROTECTION

The motorcyclist's breaths sound labored, a deep gurgling sound rising from the back of his throat.

The A in the ABCs stands for Airway management. Your character will need to make sure the path leading from the victim's mouth to their lungs is open and clear. To do this, your character will need to check for signs of obstruction or swelling. In conscious victims, signs of partial airway obstruction include noisy breathing, choking sounds, wheezing, or a suddenly hoarse voice. If your character is frantic, starting to turn blue around the lips, or fighting to breathe but making no sound, their airway is totally occluded. If they're unconscious, look for blue-tinged lips, uncontrolled drooling, and a lack of chest movement.

To open the airway, your character will need to position the victim. If they're actively vomiting, position them on their side so they won't aspirate—breathe in their vomit. Otherwise position them on their back, with their mouth open and the jaw thrust forward. If there is something in their mouth that is obstructing their breathing, your character should pull it out. Ideally, they'd do this with forceps or another tool—your character doesn't want their fingers bitten off!

> In unconscious victims, the most common cause of obstruction is the tongue falling into the back of the throat.

The trick with positioning and intubation is C-spine protection. The cervical spine, or C-spine, makes up the neck, and the portion of the spinal cord it protects is critically important to the basic functioning of the human body. If the spinal cord is severed at these levels, the diaphragm—along with every other muscle in the body—is permanently paralyzed, making it impossible for your character to breathe on their

> Victims of overdose, drownings, or head wounds are at highest risk of aspiration.

own ever again. If the victim could have broken their neck, your character needs to make sure those broken fragments don't sever the spinal cord.

Aida, no longer on the phone, holds the man's head still with her hands and thrusts his jaw forward. The gurgling sound stops, and the man's breaths sound clear.

C-spine protection requires complete immobilization of the victim's neck. To do this, your character should hold the victim's neck very still as the airway is opened and manipulated. If one is available, your character should place a cervical collar, a hard plastic collar fastened around the victim's neck to prevent movement.

> If your character doesn't have a c-collar on hand, they could improvise one using pillows or bulky jackets – anything that will keep the victim from moving their neck.

If the victim's airway still isn't open despite correct position, they will need to be intubated–a tube stuck down their windpipe to give direct access to the lungs. But unless your character is a doctor or paramedic AND they have intubation equipment with them, intubation is impossible.

If intubation fails, the Hail Mary is to perform a *cricothyrotomy*. TV shows love this procedure–a knife or needle inserted between the thin cartilage rings of the trachea to open the airway, bypassing whatever blockage is above. In reality, this procedure is rarely performed, and only by specialists, usually in the controlled setting of an OR with a patient who has anatomy that makes intubation difficult. However, the drama of an off-duty surgeon saving someone's life with a butterknife to the neck is hard to deny.

BREATHING

The next step in the ABCs is breathing. To test for breathing problems, your character should first look to see if the victim's chest is rising and falling. If they aren't breathing, but the airway is clear, your character will need to breathe for them, but don't jump straight to mouth-to-mouth! Medical professionals never touch their mouths to a patient's; they use a bag valve mask (BVM) instead. Human mouths are gross, and mouth-to-mouth is an excellent way to get a nasty infection. But if your character is alone in the field, and they don't have this equipment with them, they'll be forced to choose: risk becoming infected with a lifelong, incurable illness (like Hepatitis C), or let the victim die. What a delightful conundrum!

> A **BVM** is a football shaped inflated bag that is squeezed to force air into the victim's lungs, a process called giving breaths.

If the victim is breathing on their own,

look for signs that their breathing is insufficient, such as cyanosis, breathing that is too fast or too slow, wheezing or crackling lung sounds, and wounds to the chest. Agonal breathing–slow, gasping breaths–is a sign of imminent death.

Depending on your character's training and the equipment available, there are lots of things they can do to improve breathing, ranging from intubation and mechanical ventilation with a bag valve mask to simply administering oxygen.

> **Cyanosis** is the medical term for skin turning blue. It is first seen around the lips, nail beds, and gums.

CIRCULATION

Al checks the man's pulse by pressing a finger to the man's neck–the pulse is weak and thready, but there.

Circulation disorders include everything from bleeding wounds to acute myocardial infarctions. If blood is going where it shouldn't or isn't getting to where it should, it's a circulation problem. And yes, circulation is the *third* priority on this list. That doesn't mean your character shouldn't slap a bandage and some pressure on a spurting artery the moment they see the victim. But if it comes down to applying a tourniquet or opening up an airway, your character should always choose the airway. After all, you can lose quite a lot of blood before dying, but you can't go long without breathing.

> A **myocardial infarction** is the medical term for a heart attack.

Signs of circulation disorders include no pulse, a heartbeat that is too fast or too slow, cool and clammy skin, slow responses, confusion, or agitation. If your character has a BP cuff on them, they might notice the victim's blood pressure has dropped precipitously. And, of course, any wound gushing blood is a circulatory disorder.

> **Tachycardia** is a fast heart rate. **Bradycardia** is a slow one.

Al can see a dark patch of blood staining the victim's jeans, a stick jammed into the inside of his thigh. Al rips off a bit of the man's shirt and presses it against the wound. He considers trying to pull out the stick but decides against it. It looks really lodged in there.

Blood does not have to be gushing out on the sidewalk for the victim to be losing massive amounts of it. The victim could lose their entire body's volume of blood into their abdomen or pelvis, and your character wouldn't see anything besides

> If something is sticking out of your character's body (knife, stick, ice pick, etc.), please do NOT have your character pull it out.

maybe some bruising. That stick in the motorcyclist's thigh might be the only thing keeping him from bleeding out!

Causes of circulatory disorders range from bleeding wounds to heart attacks and heart failure. Depending on the resources your character has on hand, the most they might be able to do is to bandage the wound and put pressure on it. If the victim has lost a lot of blood and your character has the resources, they should start two IV lines–one in each arm–and give fluids to help prop up the circulatory system until blood products can be given.

The ambulance arrives and Al tells the paramedics what happened. Aida, still holding c-spine, asks what she can do to help. The paramedic tells her to continue holding the c-spine and jaw thrust while they perform a more detailed exam.

After the ABCs have been taken care of, a healthcare provider will evaluate the DEs: Disability and Exposure.

DISABILITY

One paramedic begins by assessing the victim's mental status, calling him "sir" loudly and telling him to open his eyes. The motorcyclist's eyes flutter open, then quickly close again. With Aida keeping the victim's head and neck firmly in place, the paramedic pinches his earlobes, watching him wince in pain. Al watches curiously, noticing that the victim moves his arms sometimes, but never his legs.

You'd think disability would mean that the victim has part of a leg missing or that they've chopped their fingers off. But in the primary assessment, disability means looking for severe neurologic or psychiatric changes. This can include:

- Altered mental status
- Agitation, disorientation, or delirium
    - Altered level of consciousness (Ch. 19)
    - Confusion, tiredness, or lethargy
- Convulsions
- Neurologic changes
    - Headache +/- neck rigidity
    - Paralysis
    - Uneven, dilated, or constricted pupils
- Psychiatric changes

> **Convulsions** are uncontrolled, rapid muscle contractions causing violent shaking. Colloquially, they're used interchangeably with seizures, but they're not the same thing. Convulsions are a symptom–the actual shaking. **Seizures** are an electrical storm in the brain that may or may not cause convulsions.

Emergent treatment for neurologic and psychiatric disability ranges from skilled de-escalation to emergency neurosurgery.

EXPOSURE

After the paramedics have cut off the man's clothes, they can see road rash over the left side of his body, and a few gashes on his left arm and chest. The left thigh—the one with the stick in it—is discolored and swollen.

Looking for exposure means a more thorough physical exam, looking for wounds or sources of contamination that might have been missed. To do this, your character will need to strip the victim and "log roll" them to look at their back. Since it takes too much time to undress the victim (and some injuries can be exacerbated by pulling off clothes) every emergency provider carries trauma shears—scissors sharp enough to cut through jeans or leather boots. Not all victims are a fan of having their favorite pair of jeans cut in half but missing a vital injury could be the difference between life and death.

> People who have lost a lot of blood are at risk of hypothermia, so have your character give the victim a warm blanket if possible.

Along with the paramedics, Al and Aida help log roll the still-unconscious victim onto his side, and the lead paramedic checks his back. There's a worrisome bruise emerging on his left lower back. They place a c-collar around his neck, then lay him down onto a backboard, securing him in place before lifting him onto a stretcher and loading him into the ambulance.

Once the victim is fully exposed, your character will look for signs of injury—bruises, cuts, burns, etc.—or internal bleeding. They will feel up and down the spine, looking for tenderness that might indicate a break in the vertebrae. If there is no neck tenderness—and the patient is awake and coherent—your character might remove C-spine precautions and take off the C-collar, much to the relief of the victim.

> C-collars are uncomfortable. No one likes wearing them.

While looking for exposure, your character is also looking for signs of abuse (Ch. 16), IV drug use, or sources of contamination, like pesticides or radiation. The next step is to get the victim to the hospital for further evaluation.

BREAKING DOWN A CLICHÉ: THE LONE WOLF

"I work alone."–Every fictional doctor ever.

In medicine—and especially emergency medicine—no one works alone. In the ED, your character will be swarmed by a team of doctors–attendings, fellows, residents, and interns–along with nurses, respiratory therapists, ER technicians, scribes, and students. Even in the field, medics and EMTs work in pairs, and usually have backup from firefighters and police. Fire and police usually arrive before the ambulance and make sure the scene is safe and the victim isn't stuck in a dangerous situation.

Because most emergencies are treated by a team, the medical approach to an emergency assumes that there are other people present. Many maneuvers, such as the log roll, placing a victim on a backboard, or even lifting the patient onto a gurney are simply impossible alone.

If your character is going to have to respond to a medical emergency by themselves, they need to struggle a bit. If the victim doesn't have a pulse, what do they do first: start CPR or run back to their car to grab their cell phone and call 911? What if the victim is laying on their stomach, occluding their airway, but there's a good chance that moving them will sever their spinal cord? How will your character respond if *two* victims require life-saving treatment?

In real life, these situations can feel like a nightmare. There is no right answer; only the lesser of two evils. If your character ever finds themselves in a lone rescue situation, they are going to have to make some tough choices and make them fast. Talk about a tense plot point!

> On average, it takes an urban ambulance less than 8 minutes to arrive after a 911 call. That time rises significantly in rural areas.[1]

14. SHOCK

Brenda is washing dishes when she hears her 4-year-old son Brayden cry out in pain from the living room. She rushes over to find that he's pulled her sewing machine off the table and is lying pinned beneath it on the living room floor. She pulls it off him, comforting him as he cries. He doesn't appear badly hurt, but he is sobbing and clutching his belly. Brenda scoops him into her arms and rushes to the ED.

IF YOUR CHARACTER IS IN shock, it means something has gone drastically wrong. Often, the first hint that something is wrong is a change in their vital signs.

VITAL SIGNS

Vital signs monitor your character's wellbeing. The four main vital signs are heart rate, breathing rate, blood pressure, and temperature. Weight and blood oxygen levels are also sometimes considered vital signs.

> Elevated vital signs during exertion are normal!

By the time they arrive at the Emergency Department, Brayden is no longer crying, just holding his belly and whimpering. The triage nurse listens to his heart and lungs with a stethoscope, then uses a child-sized blood pressure cuff around his arm. The nurse frowns and tells Brenda that Brayden's pulse is fast, and his blood pressure is a little lower than expected. He's taken immediately back to a room.

Vitals are measured when your character is at rest. If your character's vital signs fall within the normal range, their vital signs are considered 'stable.' Outside that range, the vitals are unstable and indicate that something may be seriously wrong. The table below gives some basic parameters for these vital signs but be aware that they may fluctuate based on age, gender, weight, and other factors.

Vital Sign	Medical Term	Units	Normal	Too High	Too Low
Blood Pressure	Blood Pressure (BP)	mmHG	Normotensive (120/80)	Hypertension (>140/90)	Hypotensive (<90/60)
Pulse Rate	Heart Rate (HR)	Beats per minute	Normal rate and rhythm (60-100)	Tachycardia (>120 BPM)	Bradycardia (<60 BPM)
Breathing Rate	Respiration (RR)	Breaths per minute	Normal rate (12-20)	Tachypnea (>25)	Bradypnea (<12)
Temperature	Temperature (T)	Degrees Fahrenheit	Normothermic (97.8- 99.1)	Febrile (>100.4°F)	Hypothermic (<95°F))

Vital signs are just that: vital. Even just one of them being too high, or too low, is an indication that something is going seriously wrong. If your character's vital signs are off, they'll feel it, whether as a racing heartbeat, trouble catching their breath, or the shakes and chills of a fever. The exception is high blood pressure, which is asymptomatic. If your character's blood pressure gets too low, they will go into shock.

> Changes in vital signs are not a diagnosis. If your character's vital signs are off, the most important question is why.

HALLMARKS OF SHOCK

The emergency department doctor arrives only a few minutes later, but Brayden is already so drowsy that Brenda has to shake him to get him to open his eyes. His hands are cold, his lips turning a bluish purple. The doctor asks what happened and examines Brayden's stomach, which seems more bloated than usual. When he presses on Brayden's abdomen, the boy screams in pain.

Shock occurs when the body's organs are not getting enough blood to survive. If your character is in shock, their pulse will quicken, and their heart may feel like it's galloping or beating irregularly. Their breaths will come fast and shallow, they will feel extremely tired and may become anxious confused, or disoriented. Their mouth and mucous membranes will feel dry as sandpaper and they won't even be able to urinate.

How shock is treated depends on what type of shock it is. There are four main types of shock: hypovolemic, cardiogenic, neurogenic, and septic shock. Let's start with the obvious: loss of blood volume.

> Low urine output = oliguria
>
> No urine output = anuria

HYPOVOLEMIC SHOCK

If your character doesn't have enough blood, they won't be able to get enough oxygen to their organs. Hypovolemic (Latin for "under volume") shock can happen because of either blood loss or fluid loss. That's right—you don't *have to* make your character bleed out to give them hypovolemic shock. But you certainly can. Since writers love making their characters bleed out, let's start by talking about the symptoms of shock caused by blood loss.

> Blood thinning medications can turn a minor injury into a life-threatening hemorrhage.

HEMORRHAGIC SHOCK

The doctor explains that Brayden is bleeding internally, which is causing his blood pressure to plummet. Most likely, he ruptured his spleen, but they won't know for sure until they do surgery, called an exploratory laparotomy, or "Ex-Lap," to find the source of the bleeding and stop it.

If you want your character to go into hemorrhagic shock, they're going to need to lose *a lot* of blood. Adults have 4-6L of blood in their body, depending on their age, weight, and gender. How your character feels will depend on both how much blood they've lost, and how quickly. The faster the blood loss, the less time the body has to adjust, and the more catastrophic the bleed will become. Medical students remember the symptoms of blood loss using the 10-20-30% rule.[1]

> Pregnant women have a higher volume of blood. Children have a smaller blood volume.

- 10% blood loss (0.5L): Your character will barely feel anything; their heart might beat a bit faster. This is about how much blood they take during a routine blood donation.

- 20% (1L): Your character will start to feel anxious and dizzy, especially when they go from lying down or sitting to standing, a phenomenon called *orthostatic hypotension*.

- 30% (1.5L): At this point, your character is in shock. They'll feel woozy, drowsy, or have difficulty focusing. Their pulse will race, and they'll start breathing fast and shallow. If someone takes their blood pressure, it will be low (<90/60).

> 1.5L of blood is a bit more than a Supersize drink from McDonald's.

- 40% (2L): Your character has exsanguinated, and they will lose consciousness. At this point, they're probably going to die.

- 50% (2.5L): They're dead, or close to it.

Big, relatively shallow arteries, like the femoral (groin), carotid (neck), or radial (wrist) arteries are good targets if you want your character to bleed out on the sidewalk. But most of the time, the real danger is internal bleeding.

If your character is going to bleed internally, they're most likely going to bleed into the thigh, pelvis, abdomen, or chest (thorax), as those are the places that can hold the most blood. Internal bleeding has a host of different causes, ranging from trauma to ulcers.

> Your character can't exsanguinate from a brain bleed – there isn't enough space inside the skull. Instead, they'll die. of brain herniation. (Ch. 19)

NON-HEMORRHAGIC

Of course, blood loss isn't the only way for your character to experience hypovolemic shock. Severe dehydration can also cause hypovolemic shock, as can copious vomiting or diarrhea. Burns, which cause large amounts of water loss from damaged skin, is another cause. So, if your character is lost in the desert without water, covered in burns, or has been sh*tting their brains out due to food poisoning, they'll be at risk of hypovolemic shock without ever spilling a drop of blood.

TREATMENT

Nurses and doctors surround Brayden. They hold him still as they start IVs in the crook of both his arms, hanging bags of fluid and placing splints to keep him from moving his arms around. Next, they take blood samples to determine Brayden's blood type and start a blood transfusion a few minutes later. A pediatric surgeon explains the risks and benefits of the "Ex-Lap" to Brenda, who agrees readily. Within minutes, Brayden is whisked off to surgery.

Hypovolemic shock is treated by giving high volume IV fluids in a process called Fluid Resuscitation. If your character's shock is not due to hemorrhage, fluid resuscitation will likely be enough. If your character has had a significant blood loss, they'll need a blood transfusion.

> O negative blood is considered the Universal Donor blood type because it lacks proteins, found on other blood types, which stimulate an immune response.

Blood transfusions don't always happen immediately–the doctors need to make sure they're giving the right blood type, using a test called a *type and screen*. Sometimes, the correct blood type has to be brought in from a blood bank. If there isn't time, your character will be given Type O blood.

OTHER TYPES OF SHOCK

Other types of shock include septic, cardiogenic, and neurogenic shock.

Cause	Blood Pressure	Heart Rate	Skin	Urine Output
Cardiogenic	Low	Fast & Irregular	Cool, pale	Low
Hypovolemic	Low	Fast	Cool, pale	Low
Neurogenic	Low	Slow	Warm, pale	Low
Septic	Low	Fast	Hot, red	Low

Cardiogenic shock occurs when the heart isn't beating properly, such as during heart failure or myocardial infarction. If your character is in cardiogenic shock, they'll have the same cool clammy skin and fast heart rate as hypovolemic shock, but the veins in their neck will become engorged as the blood flowing into the heart gets backed up. And their heart rate will be fast and irregular.

Neurogenic shock, also called Distributive Shock, occurs when the peripheral veins and arteries dilate so much that blood isn't returned to the heart. It is usually due to a spinal cord injury and is characterized by a slow heart rate and cool, clammy skin. Anaphylactic Shock, a severe type of allergic reaction, is a subtype of distributive shock.

Septic shock occurs when your character has an infection that has entered their bloodstream, causing their immune system to go haywire. It is characterized by fever, a high heart rate, and hot, flushed skin. Despite their fever, they may have *rigors*–the medical term for trembling or feeling cold despite a fever.

> While most people will have a fever, some–especially the very old and the very young–will have a low body temperature (<96.8oF). This is a bad sign.

BREAKING DOWN THE CLICHÉS:

EMOTIONAL SHOCK

A beautiful woman answers the door, her face falling as she sees two police officers instead of the man she was waiting for. The two officers share concerned looks, then gently tell her that her lover was killed. The woman screams, clutches her heart, and falls to the floor, dead.

Nothing sounds quite so romantic as dying of a broken heart. And while it seems like something out of a sappy romance novel, severe emotion *can* cause heart-attack-like symptoms. Colloquially it's called 'broken heart syndrome,' but the medical term is *Takotsubo's Cardiomyopathy.*

In this rare syndrome, extreme emotional distress sends a flood of hormones through the body so strong that it causes the heart muscle to squeeze in a highly abnormal motion, causing compromised blood flow. The symptoms look just like a heart attack–chest pain, trouble breathing, dizziness, etc. More common in women and the elderly, the exact mechanism isn't known, but it's estimated that 5% of all women diagnosed with a myocardial infarction (the medical term for a heart attack) actually suffered from this syndrome instead.

Fortunately, this condition is usually temporary and improves with medical care. Unlike what you see in movies, it's pretty rare for anyone to die from Takotsubo's Cardiomyopathy.

> While grief is the most common cause, Takotsubo's Cardiomyopathy has been triggered by domestic abuse, severe pain, car accidents, and even public speaking.[2]

'TIS BUT A SCRATCH

Spurting arterial wound? No problem. Blood soaking through a shirt and pooling on the floor? Get up and keep fighting!

Characters in movies and video games have a remarkable ability to keep fighting or running despite massive amounts of blood loss. That just isn't realistic. Remember the 10-20-30% rule? That only applies if your character is at rest. If they're needing to get their heart pumping–say by engaging in a sword fight or running away from a monster–they're going to feel that blood loss a lot more acutely.

Think about how you've felt after donating blood. Did you feel a little dizzy when you first tried to stand up? Were you told to drink a lot of water, eat some cookies, and sternly warned against trying to walk the two miles back to your house?

A blood donation is usually about 1 pint of blood–around 10% of your total blood volume. With that small amount of blood loss, you may not feel anything when you're sitting around watching television. But if you went for a run or even just a brisk walk, you'd probably feel a little breathless, maybe even dizzy. Keep that in mind when you're deciding how seriously to injure your character if you still want them to keep fighting.

> Yes, adrenaline will help your character stay on their feet. But if they're losing blood fast, adrenaline is already pumping through their system–it's the body's natural defense. It doesn't make them invincible.

15. CARDIOPULMONARY RESUSCITATION (CPR)

Caleb, a volunteer firefighter, is helping his mother, Charlotte, shovel snow out of the driveway when she collapses. Caleb runs over and shakes her, yelling for help. When she doesn't respond, he stops, takes a big breath, and exhales into her mouth, before moving to her side and beginning chest compressions. Minutes later his partner, Cody, arrives, having heard Caleb's cries for help. He dials 911, then races across the street towards the gas station.

WHAT IS CPR?

CPR stands for **Cardiopulmonary Resuscitation**. It is used only when someone has no pulse. CPR can occur anywhere: in the field, in the hospital, even in the OR. It is a core component of BLS–Basic Life Support–and can be performed on anyone, from newborn babies to the elderly.

If your character has no pulse, it means their heart isn't pumping blood to their vital organs. CPR forces blood to flow through the body. By performing chest compressions, your character is squishing and unsquishing the victim's heart, manually forcing blood through. Seem kind of gross? It gets worse. The provider performing CPR has to push really hard for it to work. The saying is that if you aren't breaking bones, you aren't pushing hard enough.

> "Found down" means your character stumbled across someone without a pulse, but they don't know how long they've been unconscious. It prevents your character from doing CPR on a corpse.

WHEN SHOULD CPR BE PERFORMED?

CPR should only be performed on someone whose heart recently stopped beating. To start CPR, your character should ensure that the victim:

- Has no pulse
- Isn't breathing
- Is unconscious and unable to be woken
- Has been "down" for a known length of time

PERFORMING CPR

1. Check for a pulse.
2. Position the character on their back with their chin tilted up to open the airway.
3. Begin compressions, counting aloud.
4. For every 30 compressions, a second person gives two rescue breaths.
    a. If your character is alone, skip the rescue breaths & continue with compressions only.
5. Continue until AED or emergency medical personnel arrives.

> Compressions should be given at a rate of 100-130 beats per minute, to the tempo of "Stayin' Alive" or the Baby Shark song if your character is a Millennial or younger.

CPR Dos and Don'ts

Do	Don't
Check for a pulse or breathing.	Perform CPR on someone who is conscious.
Call for help.	Perform CPR on someone who was 'found down.'
Move the victim away from potential hazards.	Perform CPR in an unsafe situation.
Count compressions out loud.	Push too fast or too slow.
Perform CPR on children, babies, and even pets.	Forget to modify CPR for babies, children, and pets.
Push hard.	Shy away from breaking bones.

Sound exhausting? It is—both mentally and physically. Whether done in the field or in a hospital, CPR takes a toll on both the victim and the provider.

> Performing CPR is hard. Good CPR is even harder. Many times, paramedics and doctors will differentiate "Bystander CPR" from "Effective CPR" because so many people do it wrong.

As Caleb performs compressions, he positions his hands in the middle of his mother's chest, pressing hard with the heel of his hand. He is strong, and his mother is frail; with every compression, he feels her ribs cracking beneath his hands, the broken edges of bone grinding together. Within minutes, Caleb's muscles feel like water and, despite the cold, he feels the sharp sting of sweat falling into his eyes.

CPR is exhausting, but it's also just a sustaining technique; it's rare for someone to spontaneously regain a pulse with just CPR. To get a pulse back, you need a defibrillator and/or some potent IV medications. In the field, that means an Automatic External Defibrillator.

THE AED

AED stands for **A**utomatic **E**xternal **D**efibrillator. Found in all public places, from airports and gas stations to elementary schools, AEDs are meant to be used by pretty much anyone. The AED gives verbal commands to help your character administer electric shocks and/or CPR while waiting for emergency services.

Cody returns with a bright yellow AED. Caleb sits, back, wiping sweat from his eyes as Cody unbuttons Charlotte's shirt and places the sticky pads on her chest: one above the right breast, the other on her left side. The device buzzes to life.

"Stop compressions," it commands. "Analyzing rhythm."

The AED has four basic commands.

1. Analyzing rhythm.
2. Resume CPR.
3. Shock Advised: your character will press the big yellow (or red) "Shock" button.
4. Clear: everyone must stop touching the victim to allow the AED to deliver a shock and/or analyze the heart's rhythm.

Following the AED's command, Caleb sits back on his heel. He shoves down his panic—logically, he knows the machine can't analyze his mother's heart rhythm while he's pushing on her chest, but the seconds seem to drag on forever.

"Resume compressions."

Caleb watches, panic rising as Cody takes over giving compressions. After two minutes, the AED buzzes again.

"Stop compressions. Analyzing rhythm." A few breathless seconds pass, then the AED speaks again. "Shock advised."

Caleb leans back, making sure neither he nor Cody are touching his mother, then presses the red button. "Stay Clear" the AED intones, then there's a buzz, and Charlotte's shoulders jump slightly. There's a breathless pause, then "no shock advised." Caleb check's his mother's pulse, and feels it, weak and thready beneath his fingers. Seconds later, the ambulance arrives.

Sometimes, an AED can get the victim's heart to beat again. Other times, a more targeted approach is necessary, using a combination of defibrillation, compressions, and some potent IV medications. That's where advanced cardiac life support comes in.

ADVANCED CARDIAC LIFE SUPPORT (ACLS)

When the paramedics arrive, they check for a pulse, then get straight to work. One begins intubation while the other pulls off the AED pads, replacing them with sticky pads from the defibrillator from the ambulance. The defibrillator spits out a strip of white paper with red lines–an EKG strip–which the lead paramedic reads while the other places an IV. Caleb watches them work, feeling helpless. The paramedics place his mother on a gurney and load her into the ambulance.

ACLS, provided by healthcare workers such as doctors and paramedics, is a constantly evolving system of evaluating the patient's heart rhythm, then providing defibrillation (electric shock), airway monitoring and intubation, manual compressions, and giving cardiac medications by IV. It's beyond the scope of this book to explain the complicated ACLS algorithm but know that ACLS can be performed in a healthcare setting, such as a hospital or clinic, or by paramedics in the field.

> Healthcare providers read EKG strips to determine the victim's heart rhythm.

	AED	Manual Defibrillator
Locations	General public (airports, schools, stores, doctor's offices).	Healthcare (hospital, ambulance).
Users	Anyone.	Healthcare professionals (doctors, paramedics, advanced practitioners).

	AED	Manual Defibrillator
Description	Yellow/red box with sticky pads connected by wire and three buttons: power, charge, and shock.	Box with multiple buttons and dials, monitor showing heart rhythms. May have sticky pads or metal paddles (with gel).
Monitor	Shows simple written directions on face (or does not have a monitor face at all).	Displays heart rate, breathing rate, and oxygen saturation. Prints out EKG on red-lined paper.
Sounds	Loud, monotone instructions. Hum of charging. Blaring tone before shock.	Beeping heart rate. Hum of charging. Blaring tone before shock.

AEDs and manual defibrillators are not the same things. AEDs are found in the field–in grocery stores, airports, and schools–and are meant to be used by pretty much anyone. Manual defibrillators are used only by trained medical professionals and are more customizable. Most defibrillators–automated or not–use disposable sticky pads that go on a patient's right chest and left side.

Isn't the heart on the left side of the chest? Yes. The pads are placed so that they will conduct electricity *through* the heart. In kids, they can be placed front and back, but that isn't feasible for heavy adults.

> "Code" is short for **Code Blue**. There are a bunch of different hospital codes (Code Pink, Code Orange, etc.) but Blue is the only Code anyone really pays attention to, so it's just called a Code.

ACLS IN THE HOSPITAL

In the hospital, if a patient is found to have no pulse, a Code Blue is called. When that happens, the Code Team–usually made up of residents, interns, and sometimes a respiratory therapist or nurse–arrives with the Crash Cart: a wheeled cart carrying everything the team needs. Everyone on the Code Team has a role.

1. **Team Leader**: The person running the code. Always a physician, usually a resident. Stands at the foot of the bed, reads the EKG rhythm strip, and gives orders based on the heart rhythm.

2. **Airway**: Intubates the victim, connects the BVM and gives breaths. Must be a physician, RT, or APP.

> "Push" means to inject medications through IV.

3. **Code Cart and Defibrillator:** Gathers supplies from Code Cart and administers shocks when advised by the team leader. Usually a physician, such as Junior Resident or Intern, but could also be a nurse or APP.

4. **Medication Nurse:** Starts an IV and pushes the meds ordered by the Team Leader.

5. **Recorder:** Documents every step and medication given, relays orders to a runner if additional supplies are needed.

6. **Runner:** Retrieves additional supplies.

7. **First Responder:** The person who called the Code (usually the victim's nurse). Informs the Team Leader what happened. May also act as Recorder or Runner.

8. **Compressors:** Stand on a stool and gives compressions. Medical students, nurses, and other healthcare personnel line up to help with compressions—each provider only gives compressions for two minutes to prevent tiring out.

ACLS IN THE FIELD

ACLS can also be provided by paramedics on the scene or in the back of an ambulance. Depending on the precinct, paramedics usually work in teams of two, often with one paramedic and one EMT. Firefighters trained in BLS might be on the scene to help give compressions. But sometimes, it is down to just the medic doing everything themselves while their partner drives the ambulance to the hospital.

DO NOT RESUSCITATE ORDER (DNR)

Advance directives are legally binding orders that spell out end-of-life preferences to family and medical practitioners in the event they aren't able to make those decisions when the time comes. The most famous advance directive is the Do Not Resuscitate (DNR) order.

The DNR is a legally binding order to abstain from CPR. Theoretically, if your character has a DNR and collapses without a pulse, no one will start CPR and they will be allowed to remain dead. But there's a catch. In America, we'll sue anyone for anything, particularly when it comes to healthcare, so the general practice is CPR unless proven otherwise. This mentality means the burden of proof for a DNR lies with the family or friends. The laws vary from state to state. In some places, just telling the provider that the patient has a DNR is enough; others require the actual paperwork. This is an

> DNRs aren't just for old people: anyone who doesn't like their chances of ending up in a coma after CPR should have one. I do.

excellent potential source of tension, between the family member and provider or between two family members. It can even be a source of internal struggle: neglect a loved one's explicit wishes, or allow them to die before your character's eyes? It's a horrible situation in real life—but doesn't that make for some of the best writing?

BREAKING DOWN THE CLICHÉS

There are plenty of misunderstandings about CPR and ACLS, and for good reason. There is so much potential drama there; it is literally life or death. By avoiding some of these clichés, you can keep the drama, but skip the eye rolls from everyone in the medical field.

FLAT-LINING[2]

Nurse: "We're losing them, doc!"

Aggressive monotone blare of patient monitor, which shows only a flat line

Nurse: "They're flatlining! We've lost them."

Doctor: "Not on my watch!" *Rubs paddles together* "Clear!"

Patient jerks as electricity floods his body *Tense silence. No one moves* *Patient gasps and opens his eyes, coughing. Monitor starts beeping happily*

Doctor: "Welcome back, son."

Unfortunately, that's not how it works.

First of all, that monitor over the patient's bed is not an ECG. It measures pulse rate, breathing rate, and blood pressure. If there's a flat line on that monitor, it's probably because your character disconnected themselves to walk to the bathroom.

Second, people don't jump off the table when they get a shock. There's a little jolt, and sometimes the hips and shoulders jerk, but your character isn't going to be flailing all over the place. "Clear!" means stop touching the victim—otherwise your character is going to get a nasty shock.

Most of the time, the shock is delivered through sticky pads placed on the right chest and left side, like AEDs, though some hospitals still use metal paddles. Have you ever noticed that, on TV, they rub the paddles together? Doctors really do this—but it's because they've put gel on the paddle to help conduct the electricity and are trying to spread the gel around more evenly. Rubbing dry paddles together is pointless.

> If a patient is particularly hairy, a lucky someone (usually the nurse or the med student) gets to shave them first to make sure the pads stick. EDs, ambulances, and ICUs always carry disposable razors just in case.

Third, defibrillators are not a magical cure-all. Their job is to shock the heart out of bad rhythms, the most famous of which being ventricular fibrillation. That's why they're called "deFIBRILLATors"—your character is literally shocking the heart out of fibrillation.

Finally, not all rhythms are shockable. Asystole (flat line) and PEA (irregular, flat-ish line) mean that the heart doesn't have a rhythm. If you don't have a rhythm, you can't be shocked out of it. Instead, asystole and PEA—the heart rhythms that cause flat-lining—are treated with epinephrine.

And that brings me to another common trope.

SHOT TO THE HEART[3]

Riddled with bullet holes, Sergeant Maxwell Mannly drags himself past the pile of corpses—his doing, of course—and into the Med Bay. He doesn't have much time. With trembling hands, he fills a syringe from a clear bottle labeled Adrenaline. He raises the giant needle high, then slams it hard into the left side of his chest

Nothing happens, and he crumples to the ground, unconscious

Tense silence

His eyes bolt open and he gasps in a hearty breath

Let's start with what is right about this trope: epinephrine (also called adrenaline) is the correct drug to give someone who is flatlining. It can lead to a shockable rhythm or even a normal heartbeat. Yay!

The problem is with *how* it is given. Shots directly to the heart (called intracardiac injection, or ICI) were popular in the 1960s, but quickly lost traction; ICI is no more effective than IV administration and a lot more dangerous.[4] Potential dangers include puncturing a lung or causing bleeding inside the sac surrounding the heart—all of which are potentially fatal.

Finally, if your character absolutely must give someone a shot of adrenaline straight to the heart, don't just have them stab them from the front. Intracardiac injections are exceedingly delicate procedures that you just can't perform while trying to stab through ribs and cartilage. Instead, have your character slip the needle under the ribcage, aimed at the left shoulder.

REAL TALK

Unlike what you may have seen in film and television, CPR is rarely clean, pretty, or reliable.[1] High-quality CPR is exhausting, both physically and mentally. Giving good compressions isn't just physically tiring, it means breaking the victim's bones and working up a sweat. Ultimately, CPR is sad. If a character needs CPR, it's because something has gone terribly wrong. At best, your character will need lots of diagnostics and treatments once they wake up to try and figure out why their heart stopped in the first place. Unfortunately, most will never wake up at all.

Survival after CPR is pretty rare. According to a recent study, about 29% of CPR patients achieve a return of spontaneous circulation (ROSC)–meaning their heart starts beating again.[9] However, that same study found that less than 9% survived to hospital discharge.[9]

This study showed that, even if your character's heart continues to beat, it is very likely that their brain and/or other organs were permanently damaged by lack of blood flow. One study found that only 3-7% of survivors of CPR were able to return to their previous level of functioning.[5] Another study found that more than 80% of patients admitted to ICUs after CPR were comatose.[6] The vast majority of people needing CPR will never be able to return to life as they knew it–if they wake up at all.

Misrepresentation of CPR is a problem. If people think that someone can save their life by pushing lightly on their chest for a few minutes and then–poof! –they're saved, they will choose it every time. One of the hardest–and most important–things doctors do when a patient is first hospitalized is to sit down and talk with them about what they want to do if the worst happens. At first, everyone says CPR. But when you tell them what that entails, you get to watch their expression transform from mild discomfort to outright horror. No one wants to have their ribs broken or to burden their family with medical debt. Yet many people–old, dying, or otherwise frail–still choose CPR, because they still believe in the miracle that is the Hollywood portrayal of CPR.

Talking to patients about advance directives is one of the most difficult things a physician has to do. Please don't make it worse by writing a rose-tinged view of CPR.

16. ABUSE

FIRST, A CAVEAT. WRITING ABOUT abuse is hard. Reading about abuse is hard. Writers love abusing their characters (and I mean that in both the literal and colloquial sense of the word) but often don't go far enough when acknowledging or exploring the long-term cognitive, emotional, and psychological effects of that abuse. If you choose to write an abused character or an abusive relationship, you're going to need to do a lot of research on how people react and process that sort of trauma. And this chapter isn't going to be particularly helpful in that arena; I'm not a psychologist, and I haven't trained in crisis counseling. Instead, this chapter focuses on how medical professionals identify and approach victims of abuse.

Deante is almost done with his shift at the ED, but he checks the board out of habit. There's a new name there–D. Davies, room 4.

"I'll take room 4," he tells the charge nurse. He doesn't know for sure that it's Daisy, but he has a hunch. The sweet old woman has been ending up in the ED a lot lately due to falls. He hopes that tonight, he'll be able to convince her that she needs to start using a walker.

MANDATORY REPORTERS

Medical professionals are mandatory reporters of abuse. This means that if anyone–the nurse, the doctor, even the CNA or home health aide–suspects abuse, they are legally obligated to report it to the state. Since victims of abuse are often brought to the ED or clinic for the care of their injuries, doctors have to be able to distinguish normal injuries from those caused by abuse.

> Many other professionals, including teachers, are also mandatory reporters.

As Deante pulls back the curtain walling off Room 4, he's greeted by a familiar sight. Daisy sits in the hospital bed wearing a thick cardigan over her hospital gown, her left arm cradled to her chest. Her husband, Dennis, sits beside her, holding her right hand in his. As Deandre enters the room, a grin spreads across the big man's face.

"Doctor D!" Dennis says with a smile, "good to see you."

"Good to see you too," Deante replies. Dennis always accompanies his wife to the ED—the two have been married for over fifty years and are quite inseparable. "Daisy, can you tell me what happened?"

"She fell again," Dennis replies. "I think she must have tripped on the carpet or something. Broke her fall with her wrist. I've been telling her to use that cane we got last time, but you know how she is." He squeezes Daisy's hand. "Stubborn as a mule, this one."

Sitting on the hospital bed, eyes downcast, Daisy looks anything but stubborn. Deante reaches out to inspect Daisy's wrist, but as he pulls the limb towards her, the cardigan falls open, revealing a yellowing bruise just below her collarbone. It's an old bruise—too old to be from this fall, but too new to be from the last time she came to the ED. Keeping his face neutral, he turns to Dennis.

"Would you mind stepping out of the room for a moment while I complete the exam?"

Dennis chuckles. "It's nothing I haven't seen before, Doc. Besides, you want me to stay, don't you darlin'?"

Daisy nods and Dennis squeezes her hand. Deante finishes the exam of her wrist, then tells Daisy and Dennis that he thinks it is probably broken, but she'll need an X-ray to be sure.

APPROACHING VICTIMS OF ABUSE

A medical professional's job when it comes to suspected abuse is two-fold. First and foremost, the goal is to treat the victim. That can range from prescribing antibiotics for an STD to casting a broken bone. The second is to identify any red flags for abuse and document all findings. The doctor can perform this screening using a written questionnaire or by simply having a conversation.

Deante puts in the order for the X-ray, but when the medical transporter arrives, he instructs them to bring Daisy to a different room on the way back— one on the opposite side of the ED from Room 4. The nurse notifies him when

Daisy returns from the radiology department, and he hurries to her new room. Daisy is sitting up in the hospital bed, looking confused.

"Am I in the wrong room, Doctor? Where's Dennis?"

Deante takes a deep breath. "I wanted to speak with you privately if that's all right."

One of the most important things a provider can do when assessing for abuse is to speak with the victim alone. Separating the victim from their abuser can be particularly challenging; it is common for an abuser not to want to leave the victim unsupervised. In adults, it is often appropriate for the provider to insist on speaking with the patient alone, but in children–particularly small children–doing so can be virtually impossible. For that reason, medical professionals need to be alert for red flags, both in the victim and the people accompanying them.

VICTIM RED FLAGS

Daisy doesn't meet his eyes. "I don't know. Dennis usually handles this sort of thing."

Deante settles on the metal folding chair beside her bed, then points to the bruise on her collarbone. "Daisy, can you tell me what happened?"

"I told you, I fell."

"And that's how you got the bruise? Same fall as the broken wrist?"

"Of course."

Deandre nods, even though he knows it isn't true; bruises don't start to yellow for about a week. "Do you know what caused you to fall?"

"I slipped in the shower."

"Your husband said you tripped on the carpet."

"Oh, that's right. I must have forgotten. Silly me. I really am getting old."

Red flags in a victim of abuse include:
- Inconsistent or changing story
- Injuries inconsistent with the mechanism of injury described.
- Always comes to ED with the same person (parent, partner, caregiver, etc.)
    - Often allows that person to speak for them, or frequently checks in with them

- Frequent ED visits
- Delay seeking treatment
- Fear of angering the person with them
- Makes excuses for their injuries
- Wears out-of-season, baggy, or occluding clothing (i.e., long-sleeves in summer)

PERPETRATOR RED FLAGS

Red flags for perpetrators of abuse include:

- Unwillingness to let your character speak to the provider alone.
- Exaggerated or minimal concern about victim's illness/injury.
- Controls or isolates victim.
- History of frequent ED visits with the victim.
- Strong response to negative or unwanted behaviors.
- Ridicules or criticizes victim in front of others.
- Anger and hostility towards providers.
- History of animal abuse, substance abuse, and/or unemployment.
- Emotional or financial dependence on victim.
- History of marital conflict or economic struggles.
- Personal experience of abuse/neglect.

> Due to language, economic, and cultural barriers, some people may delay care or be unable to provide a consistent story. Don't confuse cultural differences for abuse!

CHILD ABUSE

Child abuse is frighteningly commonplace—nearly 700,000 children are abused or neglected in the US each year[1]—but it is often missed by providers. Writing about child abuse is particularly hard—both emotionally and technically. I don't recommend it unless your story absolutely requires it. However, if

> Personal experience of abuse – whether as the victim or witnessing a parent inflict abuse on others – is one of the strongest predictors of becoming a perpetrator.[3]

you need to hint that a child in your story is being abused, here are some common patterns you can use.

PHYSICAL SIGNS

When assessing a child's injuries, doctors should always be on the lookout for patterns of injury that are typical for abuse. Physical Signs include:[17]

- **Bites**: Human bites are elliptical or oval-shaped, and do not tear at the skin like an animal bite would.

- **Breaks:** Kids fall down, tumble from trees, and slam their hands in doors–broken bones are a normal part of childhood. However, certain types of fractures, particularly those caused by twisting injuries, are red flags for abuse.

- **Bruises:** Again, kids fall down, so some bruises are normal, particularly along the shins and knees. However, if a child is too young to be moving on their own (<6 months), or if there are many in different stages of healing, those bruises are suspicious.

> If a child has a clotting disorder, like hemophilia, they'll bruise easily. Their parents may be wrongly suspected of child abuse!

- **Burns:** Kids touch things they shouldn't. But burns due to immersion (straight lines of burnt tissue with no drip or splash marks) and mirror image burns (burns symmetrical to both sides of the body) are suspicious.
    o Small, circular burns are suspicious for cigarette burns.

- **Ear trauma:** Cuts and bruises to the outer ear are concerning for ear pinching. A perforated eardrum is particularly suspicious for hard slaps to the side of the head.[2]

- **Hair Loss:** Patches that appear torn out.

- **Head Injuries:** Accidents happen. But if a child has a brain bleed without associated skull fracture, it is more likely to be abuse–the injury was caused by shaking the child.

- **Retinal hemorrhage**: Broken blood vessels in the eye of a small child is characteristic of child abuse. It's most commonly seen in shaken baby syndrome and can be a sign of underlying brain damage.

- **Sexual Trauma:** If a kid has any signs of genital trauma or an STI, it is abuse.

> This is true for young children. Teenagers are perfectly capable of getting STI's on their own.

A WRITER'S GUIDE TO MEDICINE

BEHAVIORAL AND EMOTIONAL SIGNS

Signs of child abuse are not limited to physical signs. Changes in their behavior, mood, developmental stage, communication, and developmental regression can all be red flags for abuse.

Behavioral clues include excessive fear or anxiety, hyperactivity, poor concentration, nightmares, sleep changes, and social withdrawal. In older children, it can mean substance abuse or self-harm behaviors. Examples of developmental regression include thumb-sucking, or a previously toilet-trained child starting to wet the bed again.

Signs of sexual abuse range from the overt—the presence of an STI in a young child—to the subtle, such as a child who talks excessively or knows too much about sexual topics. Not wanting to undress or fear of being touched during the physical exam is another sign of sexual abuse.

Sometimes, the signs can be very subtle: a child who presents with frequent, nonspecific pain, or headaches that seem to come out of nowhere. Poor hygiene, inadequately tended wounds, or even a child dressed inappropriately for the weather can all be signs of neglect.

> Neglect is the most common form of child abuse in the US.[4]

PARENTAL RISK FACTORS[5]

Of course, the child isn't the only one that can show red flags. Parental behaviors that raise questions include:

- Changing or inconsistent history of how the injury occurred
- Two guardians reciting the same story word-for-word
- Explanation that doesn't fit the mechanism of injury
- Blaming a sibling or pet.
- Delayed seeking of treatment.
- No primary pediatrician, or frequently changes pediatrician.
- Unplanned pregnancy, teen parenthood.
- Parent is a caregiver for a child with significant disabilities.

If you're writing an abusive parent or caregiver, sprinkle these details in lightly. Most abusers won't exhibit all these signs—one or two will be enough to give your readers the hint.

> Not every teen parent or caregiver for a child with disabilities is an abuser. It's a risk factor, not a certainty.

DOMESTIC VIOLENCE (INTIMATE PARTNER VIOLENCE)

Intimate Partner Violence (IPV) is both widespread and highly stigmatized. In the US, about 33% of women and 25% of men will experience IPV at some point in their lives.[6] Transgender and non-binary individuals have even higher rates; one study found that over half (54%) of transgender or non-binary individuals had experienced IPV at some point in their life.[14]

> This is what should happen. IRL, red flags are often missed or dismissed out of hand.

If your character walks into the ED with any red flags for IPV, they'll be given a screening exam–either written or oral–in a private place with no one else present. Nurses trained in crisis counseling often perform the screening, though the ED doctors should follow up if there are any positive results. The doctors should also perform a thorough physical exam, looking for characteristic injuries.

"Since you had a big fall, I need to examine the rest of you," Deante says gently. "Would you mind letting me take a look? I can bring in a nurse to chaperone if you're uncomfortable."

Daisy fiddles with her blankets. "I suppose," she says finally.

Like with child abuse, victims of intimate partner violence often come to the ED or clinic with injuries and a thinly veiled story of how they got them. Often, the abuser accompanies the victim, refusing to leave their side and providing much of the medical history. While it is normal for partners to accompany a loved one to the ED, certain characteristic injuries are red flags for IPV.

INJURIES CHARACTERISTIC OF IPV

Deante gets a female nurse to chaperone, then proceeds to examine Daisy. Her back has multiple bruises of different shades–some are red and new, others faded to a dull yellowish-green. Along her upper arms, there are small, circular bruises indicative of fingerprints, as if someone had grabbed her. As he completes the exam, Daisy doesn't speak, just stares at her lap, obeying his instructions automatically. When he's completed the exam, Deante sits back down in the chair beside the bed.

"Daisy," he says gently. "Is anyone hurting you at home?"

Types of injuries include:
- Bite marks
- Bruises in the shape of a hand or fingers

- - Multiple small, circular bruises on upper arm = grab injury
  - Finger marks along face/neck/back = slap injury.
- Circular or linear bruises
- Fingernail marks (crescent-shaped impressions, scratches, and claw marks)
- Strangulation
  - Bruises or red marks around the neck: often not present and harder to see on dark skin
  - *Petechiae* on face and neck
  - Broken blood vessels in the eye, called *subconjunctival hemorrhage*
  - Sore throat, hoarse voice, or trouble breathing

> **Petechiae** are reddish purple pinpricks-sized spots caused by the bursting of tiny blood vessels in the skin.

To avoid discovery, many abusers will avoid injuring the face, instead targeting the back of the head, chest, abdomen, and breasts. Injuries to the forearms, palms, back, legs, buttocks, and back of the head are also common, suggesting that the victim was curling up to try and protect themselves.

Intimate Partner Violence can also mean more than just physical or emotional abuse. Nearly 50% of women who were physically abused also report sexual assault.[7]

RAPE & SEXUAL ASSAULT

If your character goes to the hospital after being raped, she'll likely be seen by a Sexual Assault Nurse Examiner (SANE Nurse) who will help your character through the traumatic experience. The medical evaluation begins with a history of events—what occurred before, during, and after the incident. The SANE nurse will ask for a description of the assailant, though your character does not have to provide it. Then, if your character is willing, the SANE nurse will proceed to the physical exam.

The physical exam is often very difficult for the victim. Having recently been through a traumatic experience, letting someone else—even a medical professional—touch them can be traumatic. To minimize trauma, the exam should only be done by

> I'm using female pronouns here, but men and nonbinary people can be victims of rape too.

> The process described here depicts what should happen – not necessarily what does. Victims of rape are often intimidated, blamed, or dismissed entirely. Many victims do not bother reporting, believing that doing so would be futile.

a professional trained in working with survivors of sexual assault, such as a SANE nurse. The examiner will explain every procedure, telling your character exactly what to expect and explaining the rationale behind every procedure. They will also try to empower your character, allowing her to make every decision throughout the entire procedure, such as when/where she is touched, who is or isn't in the room, or whether the door remains open or closed.

The purpose of the physical exam is to document and treat all injuries. This includes suturing closed lacerations, removing foreign bodies, and prescribing medications to prevent pregnancy and STIs, including HIV. They may also get blood and urine tests looking for "date rape" drugs like Rohypnol and GHB.

THE 'RAPE KIT'

The evidence collection kit, colloquially known as the "rape kit," is also part of the physical exam. Your character will be asked if she wants to provide evidence. If she agrees, she will be asked to give consent for each step of the process. The evidence collected includes swabs and possibly photographs of the external genitals, anus, and vagina. It also includes fingernail scrapings and clippings, along with hair, saliva, and blood samples. If your character is still wearing the same clothes they were attacked in, those may also be collected. Evidence collection can take a long time–up to several hours. But don't worry–your character will be given as many breaks as she needs. Afterward, the evidence will be sealed and stored in a secure location or given straight to the police.

> Just because an evidence kit is collected doesn't mean it will ever be used in court or even processed. There are an estimated 100,000 untested rape kits in the US.[2]

ADULT ABUSE (ELDER ABUSE)

Adult abuse is the abuse of people over 60 and those over 18 with physical disabilities. Though rarely talked about, elder abuse is common in the US–nearly 10% of people aged 60 and older have experienced some form of abuse.[9] Adult abuse can include physical, sexual, financial, and psychological abuse. The elderly are at particularly high risk for financial abuse and neglect.

> Mandatory reporters of child abuse must also report adult abuse.

SIGNS OF ELDER ABUSE

Many signs of elder abuse are similar to that of IPV and child abuse. But due to the frail and medically complex nature of this population, there are additional signs to watch out for. These include:

- Bedsores
- Clogged/dirty urinary catheter
- Yeast infections
- Poor personal hygiene
- Unexplained bruises, burns, cuts, scars, or marks indicating restraint
- Broken eyeglasses
- Lack of medical aids (hearing aid, glasses, dentures, walker, etc.)

> If your character is confined to their bed, bedsores are sign of neglect.

SYMPTOMS CONCERNING FOR ELDER ABUSE

- Trouble sleeping
- Unexplained weight loss
- Withdraws from usual activities
- Acting agitated or violent

FOLLOW-UP

Still staring at her lap, Daisy nods. "Dennis—he gets...angry sometimes. When I forget things."

"Do you feel safe at home?" Deante asks quietly.

Daisy shakes her head. "If he knew I was telling you this..." she trails off, her voice quivering.

Deante takes a deep breath, then leans forward, putting his hand over hers. "I have to report this. I'm legally obligated. Someone will come by to interview you soon. We'll find a way to keep you safe."

Daisy blinks tears from her eyes. "Thank you."

Child abuse and adult abuse require mandatory reporting. If either type of abuse is suspected, the hospital must contact both the police and either Child Protective Services or Adult Protective Services. Your character will not be allowed to return home with their alleged abuser until a primary assessment has deemed that they are not in danger.

It's a different story for intimate partner violence. Since the victims are adults who are in full control of their faculties, they have the right to decide what is safest for them. If domestic abuse is disclosed or suspected, it is the medical provider's job to provide safety information and to go over your character's options. This can include making a safety plan, connecting them with a shelter for victims of domestic violence, or giving them the number of a domestic abuse hotline.

But just because your character has acknowledged that they are being abused does not mean that they will be able to escape their situation. Often, victims of domestic abuse are unwilling or unable to leave their abuser. Medical professionals *must* respect that choice. But that often means letting a victim go home with their abuser, knowing that it will happen again. It is one of the hardest things medical professionals have to do.

BREAKING DOWN THE CLICHÉ: ONLY MEN CAN BE ABUSERS

"OMG, my husband was being so annoying last night; he loaded the dishwasher wrong–again."

"So, what did you do?"

"I kicked him in the balls!"

Everyone laughs

First and foremost, abuse is never funny. But when aimed at men, abuse is often treated as a joke. Men who have experienced abuse by women often report feeling ashamed, unmanly, or weak.[10] And if they do try to report the abuse, they are often brushed off by police and other authorities.[10]

But there is some truth to this cliché. Women are far more likely to be abused than men and are more likely to be seriously injured or killed. Around 75% of victims of domestic violence are women, and female victims of domestic abuse are more likely to experience sustained, repeated, or severe violence.[10] More than 96% of federal prosecutions of domestic violence are against male perpetrators,[11] but the number of women being prosecuted for domestic violence is rising.[12] Women tend to lean towards non-physical abuse–such as emotional, verbal, or psychological abuse–and the injuries inflicted tend to be less severe than their male counterparts.[10]

> Abuse isn't just for straight people. 17-45% of lesbians have experienced physical abuse and upwards of 50% have experienced sexual abuse by a female partner.[15]

But the picture of your typical perpetrator gets a lot murkier when you start taking child abuse and elder abuse into account. According to a 2019 study, over 53% of perpetrators of child abuse were women.[13] Gender is not a known risk factor for perpetrators of elder abuse; most perpetrators of elder abuse are the adult children of the victim.[16]

REAL TALK

Abuse is a very real and traumatizing phenomenon; writing about abuse needs to be taken very seriously. Remember; what you're writing about is real. The most horrific, degrading, and disturbing scenarios you can imagine have happened, in real life, to someone.

Done well, writing about abuse can make survivors come to terms with their situation, can even help them feel like they're less alone. But it is very hard to do well. If abuse is central to your story and character, make sure you do your research–not only on the physical effects of abuse, but on the long-term psychological, emotional, and cognitive fallout. But if you're thinking of adding scenes of abuse just for backstory or to add depth to your character, don't. Abuse isn't something you sprinkle in for flavor.

17. DRUGS & ADDICTION

Eliza has struggled with anxiety her entire life. Recently, she started having panic attacks: episodes of intense fear that seemed to come out of nowhere. She stopped going places or seeing friends, terrified that she would embarrass herself in public. Finally, she got up the courage to see a doctor. He started her on a new medication called Xanax, a benzodiazepine medication meant to prevent the attacks. And it worked! The panic attacks went away within days of starting the new meds.

BACKGROUND

ADDICTION

ADDICTION IS A CHRONIC, RELAPSING condition characterized by the compulsive seeking of the substance despite negative consequences to your character's health, finances, and social wellbeing. It has three main characteristics.

1. Cravings
2. Compulsive use
3. Tendency to relapse

Your character could be addicted to drugs, alcohol, gambling, shopping, stealing, sex, food, exercise, video games, even drinking blood.[1] But, other than drugs, alcohol, and gambling, most of these addictions are considered 'behavioral addictions' and there isn't a lot of evidence that there is a medical basis. And while a shopping addiction may have a negative fiscal impact, it certainly doesn't cause the biological changes of alcohol or opioid addictions. For this reason, medical professionals prefer the term Substance Use Disorder.

After a few months on the Xanax, it no longer seems to be keeping the edge off Eliza's anxiety. She feels more anxious than ever. Her doctor increases her dose, then increases it again a few months later. Soon, she's taking a high dose, but it still isn't working. Her doctor says that he can't increase her dose any further, so Eliza decides to take matters into her own hands.

SUBSTANCE USE DISORDERS

Like addiction, substance use disorders are characterized by compulsive substance-seeking behavior despite significant negative consequences. It is a chronic, relapsing disease. But unlike behavioral addictions, substance use disorders (and their close cousin, gambling disorder) cause physiologic changes to the body, as well as changes to behavior and thought. In substance use disorder, the circuitry of the brain itself is changed, even after your character has stopped taking it.

> **Tolerance** means your character needs higher doses to get the same effect. **Withdrawal** is a constellation of symptoms that occur when your character, already habituated to a substance, is suddenly deprived of it.

Eliza reaches out to her nephew, who she knows deals weed on his college campus. She asks if he knows anyone who sells Xanax on the street. When he seems reluctant, she tells him not to worry, it's a prescription; her insurance is being finicky and won't pay for it this month. He agrees to help her, and a few days later, meets up with her for lunch to give her a sandwich bag full of small blue pills.

Substance use disorder is characterized by four main criteria:

1. **Impaired control**: Cravings, inability to cut down, or imbibing more than intended.

2. **Social Impairment:** Withdrawal from friends and family, making mistakes at work or school, or giving up important recreational activities.

3. **Risky use:** Use in hazardous environments (such as needle sharing) or inability to stop using despite concrete negative consequences (such as a previous overdose).

4. **Biological and Pharmacological changes:** Exhibiting tolerance or withdrawal.

Your character doesn't need to meet all four criteria, but they should be experiencing more than one for a diagnosis of a substance use disorder.

When Eliza's sister finds out what Eliza asked her son to do, she is furious. Eliza promises not to contact him again. But when her supply of meds begins to dwindle, she becomes increasingly anxious. She tries to refill her prescription, only to be told that she is two weeks too early. Eliza tries to space out the meds, but she always ends up needing more. When she has a panic attack at work, she gives up and calls her nephew back. He procures another bag but tells her that this has to be the last one. He was caught with marijuana on campus and is now on academic probation. The smallest misstep and he could be expelled.

Substance Use Disorders are a class of disorders, specific to the substance being abused.

ALCOHOL

More than 85% of American adults have drunk alcohol at some point in their lives.[3] And while not all alcohol use is bad, nearly 15 million people suffer from Alcohol Use Disorder.[3]

ALCOHOL INTOXICATION

In an attempt to make her pills stretch, Eliza starts drinking vodka before bed. She's not a drinker–she's never really liked the taste of alcohol–but she's figured out the formula to get her to sleep: two shots of vodka and one little blue pill, then she sits in front of the television until she starts to feel woozy. Then she stumbles upstairs and falls asleep without bothering to crawl under the covers.

You're a writer, so I'm going to assume you've experienced the effects of alcohol at some point in your life. In case you haven't, here's a list:

- Mood changes: Euphoria, excitement, tearfulness
- Mood swings and emotional outbursts
- Stumbling and feeling clumsy
- Confusion
- Poor judgment
- Memory loss
- Nausea
- Observable signs
    o Reddened skin, flushed face
    o Slurred words

> The medical word for mood swings is **emotional lability.**

- Impaired attention and memory
- Unsteady gate, poor coordination
- Sleepiness
- Abrupt eye movements (*nystagmus*) and slow pupil dilation.

The lack of coordination that leads to stumbling, slurred words, and an inability to touch your finger to your nose during the drunk test is called *ataxia*. It is caused by alcohol's negative impact on the part of the brain that coordinates movement, called the cerebellum.

> Blackouts are caused by your character's brain's temporary inability to form new memories due to alcohol. The medical term is **temporary anterograde amnesia.**[4]

ALCOHOL MISUSE

There are a few different types of alcohol misuse. Colloquially, they are often used interchangeably, but there are important medical differences.

- **Alcohol Use Disorder (AUD):** A substance use disorder characterized by a combination of impaired control, social impairment, risky use, and biological changes.

- **Alcoholism:** A severe form of Alcohol Use Disorder characterized by physiologic changes: tolerance, dependence, and/or withdrawal.

- **Binge Drinking:** The tendency to drink a lot at one time. For men, this is five drinks in less than two hours; for women, it is four.[3] While binge drinking is not a diagnosis, it is a pattern of alcohol use that means your character is more likely to develop Alcohol Use Disorder at some point in their lives.

Before her office's annual Christmas party, Eliza takes an extra dose of her Xanax. After a few shots, she's dancing on the bar. The last thing she remembers is tripping on her heels and falling into the office hottie's arms. She wakes up the next morning on a coworker's couch–not the hottie, but the austere office secretary, who let her crash on her couch after she couldn't articulate her address for a taxi home.

> Mixing drugs is particularly dangerous.

OVERDOSE

Overdose with alcohol–also called alcohol poisoning–is dangerous and potentially life-threatening. The severity of alcohol poisoning depends on your character's blood alcohol level (BAC): the higher the BAC, the worse the symptoms. But there isn't one standard dose of alcohol that will always lead to a particular BAC; the required dose varies greatly with age, gender, body composition, tolerance, speed of drinking, and concurrent drugs or medications, among other things.

If your character has overdosed on alcohol, they may:

- Act confused or lethargic
- Be sleepy, or difficult to wake up
- Vomit
- Breathe irregularly or too slowly
- Have a slow or erratic heartbeat
- Have seizures
- Feel cool to the touch (low body temperature)

> BAC & Intoxication[5]
>
> < 0.08 = mild effects
>
> 0.08-.16 = mild impairment
>
> 0.16-0.3 = severe impairment (blackouts)
>
> 0.3-0.4 = life threatening
>
> >0.4 = comatose & death

Alcohol is cleared by the liver at a constant rate. The only cure for alcohol poisoning is time. If your character is taking care of someone who has alcohol poisoning, the only medically sound thing to do is to position them on their side so that they won't choke on their own vomit and call 911. Old wives' tales, like making the character drink coffee or telling them to go for a walk, don't help and can make things worse.

At the hospital, the doctors will give supportive treatment, draw labs to figure out your character's BAC, then give fluids and vitamins through an IV. If your character is unconscious or having trouble protecting their airway, they will be intubated and placed on a ventilator.

One thing they probably won't do is pump their stomach or give activated charcoal.[6] Alcohol is absorbed rapidly from the stomach—unless your character was drinking recently (as in, within the last hour or so), there won't be anything in there to pump. The alcohol is already in their bloodstream and making them vomit only increases the risk of aspiration.

> The medical term for pumping the stomach is a **gastric lavage.**

WITHDRAWAL

Alcohol withdrawal is one of the few withdrawal syndromes that can be life-threatening. However, most people experience only mild withdrawal. If your character has mild withdrawal, they may experience anxiety, sweating, headache, nausea/vomiting, difficulty sleeping, and a tremor in

> Withdrawal is not the same thing as a hangover. **Hangovers** are due to overconsumption of alcohol at one time and does not indicate dependence.

their hands. Mild symptoms like these start within six hours of the last drink and resolve within 48 hours. However, not all withdrawal syndromes are this mild.

Alcohol Withdrawal Seizures

Alcohol withdrawal seizures can start anywhere from 2-12 hours after the last drink. Withdrawal seizures are generalized tonic-clonic seizures, meaning your character's whole body will shake. They're scary to watch, but they generally aren't immediately life-threatening unless they last for more than 5 minutes. They are more common in people with longstanding, chronic alcoholism; once your character has had one withdrawal seizure, they're more likely to have them again.

> Alcoholic Hallucinosis and Alcohol Withdrawal Seizures are not the same thing as Delirium Tremens.

Alcoholic Hallucinosis

Alcoholic hallucinosis occurs when your character begins to hallucinate within 12-24 hours after their last drink. The hallucinations are usually visual, but they can also be auditory or tactile. If your character is experiencing alcoholic hallucinosis, they will *know* they're hallucinating, and will probably be terrified. But their vital signs will remain stable, they won't be confused or delirious, and they won't be in imminent danger.

Delirium Tremens

In contrast, Delirium Tremens–the DTs–is a life-threatening withdrawal syndrome. Delirium Tremens begins around 48 hours after the last drink and lasts anywhere from 1-5 days. It begins with a racing pulse, fast breathing, sweating, tremors, and anxiety. Your character will become extremely confused and will begin to have generalized, tonic-clonic seizures. They will hallucinate but, unlike alcoholic hallucinosis, they won't realize what they're seeing isn't real. The mortality rate of Delirium Tremens is as high as 37% if your character doesn't get treatment.[15]

If your character is undergoing alcohol withdrawal complicated by seizures, hallucinosis, or the DTs, they'll be admitted to the hospital for monitoring and treatment. The doctors will give your character a long-acting benzodiazepine, along with fluids, vitamins, and sugar to prevent complications.

> The IV bag given to withdrawing alcoholics is full of vitamins and sugar. It's nicknamed the **banana bag** due to its yellow color, which it gets from the vitamin Thiamine.

PREVENTING RELAPSE

In the US, the main strategy for preventing relapse in alcohol abusers is to promote abstinence, a healthy lifestyle, and participation in support groups such as Alcoholics Anonymous. Some medications can also help, such as Naltrexone, Antabuse, and Acamprosate.[11] While these medications are FDA-approved to treat alcohol abuse, many practitioners still don't offer these options.

> AA's structure as an anonymous organization makes it very difficult to study, as scientists can't reliably track attendance and recovery.[10]

OPIOIDS

Originally intended as medications to relieve acute pain, opioids have exploded as a drug of abuse, due in large part to the pharmaceutical and medical industry turning a blind eye to the dangers of chronic opioid use. Since 1999, the prevalence of heroin and heroin use disorder has doubled, while the number of deaths from prescription opioids has quadrupled.[7] In 2019, an estimated 1.6 million people suffered from Opioid Use Disorder, and over 70,000 died of an overdose.[20]

> It's estimated that 75% of opioid addictions started with prescription opioids.[7]

TYPES

Opioids can be found as prescriptions or as illicit street drugs; either kind can be abused.

Drug	Morphine Equivalents
Morphine	1
Codeine	0.3
Hydrocodone	1
Oxycodone	1.5
Methadone	3
Heroin	2-5
Buprenorphine	40
Fentanyl	50-100
Carfentanil	10,000

- **Opium:** The original opioid, derived from poppies, opium has been used as a medicinal and recreational drug for millennia.

- **Heroin:** A derivative of morphine, heroin is an injected street drug.
    - Comes in 3 main forms: black tar, brown powder, and white powder

- **Prescription Opioids:** Morphine, Codeine, Hydrocodone, Oxycodone, Fentanyl.[6]
    - Opioids for Long-Term Use: Buprenorphine, Methadone, Tramadol.
        - Less addictive
        - Treat opioid addiction and chronic pain.
    - Opioid Antagonist: Naloxone, treats opioid overdose

> The strength of opioids is based on its morphine equivalents. Codeine is 1/3 the strength of morphine; Methadone is 3x as strong. Carfentanil, an elephant tranquilizer often found laced in heroin or cocaine, is 10,000x stronger than morphine.[7]

INTOXICATION

No matter the type of drug ingested, the effects of opioid intoxication are similar, namely euphoria—or a feeling of well-being—coupled with drowsiness. Other signs include:

- Difficulty staying awake
- Slurred speech
- Slow breathing

OVERDOSE

An opioid overdose is a life-threatening emergency; every day, 128 people die of opioid overdose in the US alone.[21] Because opioids depress the brain's drive to breathe, the most dangerous effect of an opioid overdose is that your character will stop breathing. Observable signs of opioid overdose include

- Very slow or absent breathing
- Stuporous or unarousable
- Constricted pupils ("Pinpoint pupils")
- Pale, clammy skin

> Higher morphine equivalent opioids, such as Fentanyl, present a higher risk of accidental overdose.

> **Cyanosis**–pale or blue-tinged skin–is a sign that your character is not getting enough oxygen.

- Cyanosis of fingers and around the mouth
- Slow heart rate

Opioid overdose is treated with an antidote called Naloxone (brand name Narcan), which reverses the effect of other opioids in minutes. Naloxone works fast and can be administered by almost anyone—a fellow user, a friend, even a child. Naloxone only lasts for about an hour and a half, but if your character is fully recovered in that time—and they don't have any other intoxicants on board—they don't need to go to the hospital.

> As part of the fight against the opioid crisis, public health officials are trying to make Naloxone accessible and easy to use for everyone – especially addicts!

WITHDRAWAL

Withdrawing from opioids is a notoriously horrible experience. It isn't life-threatening the way withdrawal from alcohol is, but some people say they'd rather die than endure opioid withdrawal.

Opioid withdrawal begins anywhere from 6-30 hours after the last dose.[8] At first, your character will feel irritable and anxious. In addition to cravings, they'll have muscle aches, sweating, and trouble sleeping despite feeling tired. But they'll also have overactive bodily functions: teary eyes, runny nose, sweating, yawning, and piloerection, the medical term for goosebumps.

> The term "cold turkey" is believed to have risen from the tendency towards goose flesh during opioid withdrawal.[8]

Symptoms peak around 72 hours after the last dose; at this point, your character will feel like they have a bad stomach flu, with fevers, chills, nausea, vomiting, and diarrhea.[8] They won't be able to sleep, will feel restless or agitated and may develop a tremor in their hands. Everything—their muscles, their bones, their intestines—will hurt, and the cravings for the opioids will become nearly unbearable.

Withdrawal symptoms can last for up to a month, though the first week is usually the worst. Though not life-threatening, opioid withdrawal is often managed on an inpatient basis[9]—either at a hospital or detox facility—because it is so unpleasant.

> People who are incarcerated often have to go through opioid withdrawal without medical support.

PREVENTING RELAPSE

To prevent relapse, your character may elect to undergo rehabilitation at

> Methadone clinics can be public or private, and the level of personalized care provided varies greatly.

a methadone clinic. There, your character will work with doctors, nurses, and therapists who specialize in treating addiction. They'll be provided with counseling and behavioral therapy, as well as medication-assisted treatment such as long-acting opioids that don't give a high, like Methadone or Naltrexone. These drugs will help your character stay off the dangerous opioids by reducing cravings and withdrawal symptoms. The medical professionals will also help your character implement lifestyle and behavioral changes that will (hopefully) help them stay off the drugs for good.

But to get this treatment, your character will need to show up to the clinic regularly for their dose of methadone. They'll need to jump through insurance loopholes, massive amounts of paperwork, strict scheduling, and intensive drug testing. Your character may be trying their best to stay clean, but in the end, they may find it easier to go back to using.

> While it is possible to get a high from methadone, it is nearly impossible to do so through a methadone clinic, as the doses are low and carefully monitored.[18]

CANNABIS (MARIJUANA)

STREET NAMES
Pot, Weed, Dope, Ganja, Grass, MJ.

TYPES
Sativa (high THC), Indica (high CBD), hybrid (equivalent THC/CBD)
- THC = Tetrahydrocannabinol = Psychoactive component, produces a "high"
- CBD = Cannabidiol = Minimally psychoactive, does not produce "high"

MEDICAL USES
Medical marijuana is used to treat a variety of conditions, ranging from glaucoma to muscle spasms. There's still a lot of research that needs to be done in this field, but there is mounting evidence for using medical marijuana to treat chronic pain, seizure disorders (epilepsy), and side effects of cancer treatments, such as nausea/vomiting and appetite loss. Currently, the only FDA-approved use of medical marijuana is for the treatment of two rare forms of childhood epilepsy.

> If your character uses cannabis frequently, they could get **Cannabis Hyperemesis Syndrome**–aka a bunch of vomiting.

> CBD can be purchased in drugstores across the US.

INTOXICATION:

- Mood changes (euphoria, anxiety, relaxation)
- Change in perception (slowed time, increased tactile sensitivity)
- Impaired judgment
- Hunger/cravings
- Social withdrawal
- Delusions (usually paranoid) and hallucinations (high dose)
- Dry mouth
- Observable changes:
  - Redness in the whites of the eyes (*conjunctival erythema*)
  - Slurred speech
  - Poor coordination

OVERDOSE

Severe intoxication with cannabis is super rare. If your character is getting severe symptoms, it might be because their pot was laced with something stronger (usually cocaine).

WITHDRAWAL

- Only occurs after stopping heavy use.
- Symptoms include irritability, depression, insomnia, nausea, and loss of appetite.

> Contrary to stoner lore, it is possible to withdraw from marijuana.

HALLUCINOGENS & DISSOCIATIVE DRUGS

Hallucinogens and dissociative drugs are classes of drugs that—you guessed it—make you hallucinate. Intoxication often lasts for hours and does not result in withdrawal.

TYPES

- **LSD**: Acid, Dots, Mellow Yellow.
- **Phencyclidine:** PCP, Angel Dust.
- **Psilocybin:** Magic mushrooms, shrooms.

INTOXICATION

- **LSD:** Intoxication lasts 6-12 hours.
    - Perceptual changes (intensified colors and sensations, synesthesia)
    - Rapid and extreme shifts in emotion

Time Distortion

- Hallucinations
- Observable changes
    - Increased BP and heart rate
    - Sweating
    - Nausea

> **Synesthesia** = altered modes of sensation, such as hearing colors and seeing sounds.

PCP: Intoxication lasts 4-6 hours (dose-dependent)

- Agitation, belligerence, impulsivity
- Depersonalization (Out of body experience)
- Impervious to pain
- Superhuman-seeming strength
- Extreme aggression
- Noise sensitivity
- Hallucinations, psychosis
- Observable changes
- Rapid, involuntary eye movements (*nystagmus*)
- Pinpoint pupils
- Poor coordination
- Muscle rigidity
- High blood pressure and heart rate
- Seizures

> Someone on PCP can quickly become extremely violent. Since they don't feel pain, they take some ridiculous risks, like jumping off buildings or running through glass doors.

> Ketamine is a short-acting version of PCP.

Psilocybin: Intoxication lasts 4-6 hours

- Hallucinations
- Visual distortions (intense colors, halos, etc.)

> Psilocybin is currently being evaluated as a treatment for a variety of medical conditions, including depression and PTSD.

- Depersonalization
- Muscle weakness
- Rapid shifts in mood (often between euphoria and anxiety)
- Nausea, vomiting, or dizziness
- Observable Changes
    - Poor coordination
    - Yawning
    - Dilated pupils

WITHDRAWAL

For most hallucinogens, there is no withdrawal. The exception is PCP. If your character is withdrawing from PCP, they may feel depressed, irritable, anxious, or restless. They'll have little energy but will have trouble sleeping. Your character may become violent while withdrawing from PCP.

SEDATIVES AND ANXIOLYTICS

Sedatives and anxiolytics are drugs that depress brain activity. Alcohol and opioids are both types of sedatives, but since I already discussed them *ad nauseam*, I'm going to focus on two classes of prescription sedatives that are commonly abused: barbiturates and benzodiazepines.

TYPES

Both barbiturates and benzodiazepines are controlled substances, meaning that they are highly regulated due to the potential for their abuse.

- **Barbiturates**:
    - Treats: Headache, insomnia, seizures.[12]
        - High dose used to induce therapeutic coma (Ch. 19)
    - Prescription: Amobarbital (Amytal), Pentobarbital, Phenobarbital,
    - Street Names: Barbs, Blockbusters, Goofballs, Yellow Jackets[13]
- **Benzodiazepines ("Benzos")**
    - Treats: Anxiety, panic, insomnia, seizures, anesthesia induction

- Prescription: Alprazolam (Xanax), Clonazepam (Klonopin), Lorazepam (Ativan)
- Street names: Candy, Downers, K, K-pin, Sleeping Pills, Tranks[13]

INTOXICATION

Sedative intoxication is characterized by feelings of drowsiness and relaxation. It also results in poor coordination and an unsteady gait, slurred speech, confusion, mood swings, inappropriate behavior, and impaired judgment. If your character is looking at someone who is using benzos or barbiturates, they'll notice that their pupils will be wide and dilated.

> Benzo/Barbiturate intoxication looks a lot like alcohol intoxication; on a molecular level, all three work in similar ways.

After the Christmas party, Eliza's boss calls her into the office. He informs her that her behavior lately is unacceptable. She replies that she just had too much to drink at the party, but he waves her off. He's noticed that her pupils are always dilated at work, that her speech sometimes slurs, and she's clumsier than usual. He doesn't know what is going on with her, but it needs to stop, or she'll be fired.

OVERDOSE

At high doses, sedatives depress your character's drive to breathe. Their breathing will become shallow and slow, their skin cool and clammy, and their eyes will dilate. They will become less and less responsive, until they slip into a coma, stop breathing, and die.

If your character overdoses on barbiturates or benzos, the doctors will focus on supportive treatment: giving fluids, maintaining blood pressure, and monitoring their level of consciousness closely.[14] If your character loses consciousness or stops breathing, they'll be intubated and placed on a ventilator. If benzos were the main ingestion, doctors can give a medication called Flumazenil, which reverses benzodiazepine intoxication. But beware; Flumazenil can cause immediate withdrawal!

WITHDRAWAL

Horrified that her boss noticed changes in her behavior, Eliza decides to flush the rest of her Xanax down the toilet.

Along with alcohol, benzodiazepines and

> If your character has been prescribed high dose benzodiazepines and decides to quit taking them, they will likely begin to withdraw.

barbiturates are the only classes of drugs for which withdrawal can be fatal. And your character could become dependent on these medications even if they are taking them as prescribed. If your character is withdrawing from sedatives, they may experience:

- Sweating
- Dry mouth
- Fast heart rate and/or palpitations
- Hand tremors
- Nausea, vomiting, and decreased appetite
- Abdominal Pain
- Trouble sleeping and nightmares.
- Sensitivity to light (*photosensitivity*) and sound (*hyperacusis*).
- Ringing in their ears.
- Feeling restless, unable to sit still, or twitching
- Depression
- Severe anxiety (*Rebound Anxiety*)
- Seizures
- Delirium
- Hallucinations, delusions, or illusions.
- High blood pressure
- Dilated pupils

> **Palpitations** are a feeling that the heart is beating irregularly or too strongly.

> Untreated, 20-30% of people experiencing benzodiazepine withdrawal will have at least one seizure.2 That number jumps to 75% for barbiturates.16

That night, Eliza can't sleep. At first, she tells herself it's just anxiety, that she isn't used to sleeping without her Xanax. But her heart is pounding in her chest, and she feels so nauseated that she vomits into her bedside bin. Her mouth is dry as sandpaper, yet she's sweating through her pajamas. As the first gray light of dawn filters through her window, she can't sit still any longer. She leaps to her feet and begins to pace. The light, faint as it is, is like a knife behind her eyes, and the sound of her bare feet on the floor rings oddly.

> **Immediate withdrawal** from benzos is characterized by anxiety or insomnia that occurs within hours of the last dose.

Minor symptoms of withdrawal from barbiturates begin within six hours of the last dose and can last around five days. Acute benzodiazepine withdrawal begins within a few days of the last dose and can last anywhere from 5-28 days.[16] Protracted withdrawal–a milder form of withdrawal that affects 10-25% of benzo users–can last for up to a year.[16]

After two days of escalating nausea, sweating, and anxiety so severe Eliza wants to scratch off her skin, she calls her psychiatrist to ask for a refill. He asks what happened, and when she reluctantly tells him, he insists she be admitted directly to the hospital.

Withdrawal from benzodiazepines is treated with long-acting benzodiazepines like Diazepam.[14] Withdrawal from barbiturates is treated with phenobarbital.[14] Yup, sedative withdrawal is treated by giving your character sedatives.

Eliza drives herself to the hospital, where she is admitted for monitoring. She's started on IV fluids and a medication that the doctors tell her is a longer-acting cousin of Xanax. She still feels awful–anxious and sweaty–but it isn't quite so severe. After a few days of the benzodiazepine taper, she's switched to oral medications and discharged to an outpatient rehab facility.

The point of treatment is to give your character a lower dose of a long-acting version so that they don't feel the acute effects of withdrawal, then slowly taper them off. Detoxification tapering is a fine-tuned system that requires close monitoring. If your character is stable, dependable, and motivated to detox, AND if they have all the necessary social supports in place, they can go through the detoxification program at home, by enrolling in an outpatient treatment program. Otherwise, they'll need to be admitted to a detox center or even a hospital.

STIMULANTS

Stimulants are drugs that increase energy and alertness. Prescription stimulants such as dextroamphetamine (Adderall) are used to treat ADHD and narcolepsy. Methamphetamine and Cocaine are street drugs used as "uppers." Caffeine and nicotine are also stimulants, though their effects are much milder.

TYPES
Amphetamines:

- Medical Uses: Treat ADHD & Narcolepsy
- Prescription: Dextromethorphan (Adderall), Methylphenidate (Ritalin)
- Street Names: Meth, Speed, Crank, Ice, Bennies

Cocaine
- Medical Uses: None
- Street names:
    - Cocaine (Powder): Blow, Coke, Snow
    - Crack Cocaine (Smoked): Candy, Grit, Rocks, Sleet

> While there are no current legal uses for cocaine, coca leaves are commonly used in Peru to prevent and treat altitude sickness.

INTOXICATION

- Mood changes (euphoria, increased energy, restlessness, irritability, paranoia)
- Racing thoughts
- Chest pain or palpitations
- Hallucinations
- Impaired judgment
- Observable changes
    - Increased body temperature, heart rate, and blood pressure
    - Dilated pupils
    - Increased sweating
    - Fast speech, increased body movement
    - Hand tremor
    - Strange eye movements (*nystagmus*)

Sudden death is a side effect of stimulants, particularly cocaine, as intoxication can cause sudden cardiac arrest, stroke, or a tear in the lining of the aorta, called an aortic dissection.

WITHDRAWAL

Withdrawal from stimulants comes in the form of a post-use crash: drowsiness and exhaustion coupled with depression, a bad mood, and cravings. Sometimes, the depression can be so severe that your character may consider suicide.

> A stroke caused by cocaine use is nicknamed a "coke stroke" by ED providers.

BREAKING DOWN THE CLICHÉ: DATE RAPE DRUGS

"This drink must be high in molest-erol because it makes me want to rub myself all over you."

Unfortunately, there is an entire class of illicit drugs whose primary use is to make a victim sleepy, forgetful, and unable to fight back. These are considered date rape drugs, the most popular of which are Rohypnol, Gamma-hydroxybutyrate (GHB), and Ketamine.

- **Rohypnol:**
    - Street names: Roofies, Roche, La Rocha, Rope, Mexican Valium, Forget Pill, Mind Erasers.
    - Legal in many countries, including Mexico, as a treatment for anxiety.

> Legal Rohypnol is now sold with a bright blue dot at the center, which colors or clouds drinks so your character will know their drink was messed with.

- **GHB (Gamma-hydroxybutyrate):**
    - Street Names: Easy Lay, Gamma10, Liquid G, Cherry Meth.
    - Can easily be synthesized at home.[17]

- **Ketamine:**
    - Street names: Special K, Vitamin K, Kit Kat, Purple.
    - Basically fast-acting PCP.
    - Can result in agitation and violence.

INTOXICATION

Intoxication with date rape drugs often looks very similar to severe alcohol intoxication; for that reason, date rape drugs are often slipped into alcoholic beverages. If your character has been drugged, they may feel as if they are too drunk given how much alcohol they've had. They may also experience:

- Euphoria and increased sexual appetite.
- Blurry vision.
- Weakness.
- Inability to remember what happened while drugged or a feeling of lost time.
- Observable signs:

- Sleepiness, confusion, or sedation: can lead to coma and death in overdose.
- Ataxia: Poor coordination, slurred words, trouble walking.

If your character ingests a date-rape drug, they'll show signs of slowed brain function, called CNS depression. Their heart rate and breathing will slow, their body temperature will decrease, and their blood pressure will drop. If given too high of a dose, your character could slip into a coma or stop breathing altogether.

REAL TALK

The opioid epidemic is a very real public health crisis in the US. Millions of people are addicted, and tens of thousands of people die every year. The causes of the epidemic are diverse and multifactorial, ranging from over-prescription and PR campaigns downplaying the dangers to the economic recession.[20] It's way more complicated than I can do justice talking about here. But I do want to point out one thing.

People with addiction are people first. They can break their leg, burst an appendix, or have painful cancer metastases. If your character has a history of addiction AND an acute source of serious pain (i.e., surgery, a broken bone, or end-of-life pain) doctors *should* prescribe opioids; it's basic Medical Ethics 101.

But it doesn't always happen in the real world; doctors get jaded. If someone has a history of substance use–particularly if they're female or BIPOC–doctors are more likely to undertreat their pain or write it off as a "drug-seeking behavior." But if that person has a major, acute injury, they should receive the same treatment as someone without a history of addiction, with the addition of a referral to a pain specialist who will help them taper off once the time is right.

> If the person with the addiction doesn't want the opioids, that is also their right. Doctors shouldn't force opioids on anyone either.

18. ENVIRONMENTAL EMERGENCIES

Ever since they were kids, Finn and Felicity dreamed of through-hiking the Pacific Crest Trail, known to hikers as the PCT. They spent the last year training, and now are ready to embark on their 2,650-mile hike from the border of the southernmost tip of California all the way to the Canadian border. They set off from the Southern Terminus with their backpacks fully stocked and their hopes high. As they walk, Finn reveals that his cat, Princess Diana, bit him on the arm last night, puncturing skin. When he pulls up his sleeve Felicity can see redness surrounding the wound and streaking up his arm. Annoyed that her idiot brother didn't tell her about this injury earlier, she turns him around and marches him straight back to the car.

ANIMAL BITES

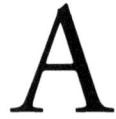

Animal bites can range from a mild annoyance to a life-threatening emergency. The severity of the bite depends on several factors, particularly the animal doing the biting and the location and depth of the bite.

CAT BITE

Cat bites are notoriously nasty; over 80% of cat bites become infected[1]. For this reason, cat bites are *not* sutured closed, as this encourages bacterial growth. If the bite broke skin, your character is going to need antibiotics. Once the red streaks show up, indicating the possibility that the infection has moved to the blood, those antibiotics will need to be given IV.

Felicity drags her brother to the doctor, who promptly diagnoses him with 'Cat Bite Cellulitis.' He's prescribed IV antibiotic infusions, which he has to get twice daily for ten days. Finn is furious at Felicity for postponing their trip, but the doctor reminds him that she probably saved his life.

> Cat scratches can also become infected with bacteria, requiring antibiotics.

DOG BITE

Most of the injury from dog bites comes not from infection, but the mechanical biting, shaking, pulling, and tearing that occurs during the bite itself. Because dog mouths are surprisingly clean (relatively speaking!), dog bites can be stitched shut and treated with oral antibiotics. Your character will also need a tetanus shot, and possibly rabies vaccine if the bite was unprovoked.

> Dog bites to the hand are not stitched closed.

BAT BITE

The bad thing about a bite from a bat is that your character won't know they've been bit. Why is that a bad thing, you ask? Because bats carry rabies, and it's virtually impossible to know you've been bitten. And since rabies is 100% fatal once symptoms show up, it is imperative that anyone who could possibly have been bitten receive treatment *before* they have a chance to show symptoms. The general wisdom is that if your character wakes up with a bat in their house, assume they were bitten and will need prophylaxis. Rabies prophylaxis includes a series of five shots—one shot of immunoglobulins given at the bite site and four serial vaccinations—given over two weeks.

> Rabies vaccines are given in the upper arm—not straight into the abdomen, as was done pre-1980s.

SNAKE BITE

The key danger in a snake bite is the venom. In the US, coral snakes and pit vipers (rattlesnakes, copperheads, water moccasins), are the primary dangers. If your character is bitten by a snake, they'll have pain and redness around the fang marks. Don't bother making a tourniquet (unless the hospital is more than three hours away) or cutting open the wound. And please don't have your character suck out the venom; human mouths are disgusting, and you're more likely to give them an infection than to remove any venom. Instead, have your character keep the injured limb above the level of the heart, keep their heart rate low—no running for the car—and get them to the hospital ASAP. Catch and kill the snake if possible—this will help doctors identify which antivenin to give—but don't waste a lot of time doing so.

> 25% of pit viper strikes do not contain venom.[1] These "dry strikes" are a great opportunity to add tension and uncertainty, but still allow your character to survive.

> Signs of severe envenomation include severe local pain, bruising, blood-tinged spit, low blood pressure and tiny purple dots over the skin, called petechiae.

Once at the hospital, your character will be given the antivenom and be monitored for dangerous sequelae, such as muscle breakdown, blood clots, bleeding, and shock. Serum sickness–an immune reaction to the venom–may cause an allergy-like reaction, with hives, fever, and painful, swollen joints. The more severe your character's symptoms, the more vials of antivenin they will need.

SPIDER BITE

Like snakes, most spider bites are harmless and will only cause a little bit of itching and redness at the site of the bite. The exceptions, of course, are the Brown Recluse and the Black Widow.

The bites of Brown Recluse spiders do not hurt immediately, but over the next several hours, can cause an ulcerating lesion at the bite site that can cause the surrounding tissue to die. It's treated with an antibiotic and–if the wound is severe–surgery to cut out the dead tissue. Black Widow spider bites hurt and swell immediately. Your character will have muscle cramping, belly pain, nausea, severe high blood pressure, and may even end up in a coma. But even the most severe bites are rarely fatal.

> The medical term for tissue death is **necrosis**.

Spider bites are very hard to diagnose, especially if your character didn't see and trap (not smush) the spider that bit them. There are lots of opportunities here for missed diagnoses here (plot point!). Not only due to bites by the wrong type of spider, but because of medical conditions that can mimic these spider bites. Diabetic ulcers, pressure ulcers, and skin infections can be mistaken for Brown Recluse bites; the abdominal pain caused by black widow bites can be mimicked by peritonitis, a potentially fatal infection.

> **Harmless Wolf Spiders are often mistaken for Brown Recluse.**

After Dan has finished his course of antibiotics, he and Felicity repack their backpacks and return to Campo and the trailhead of the PCT. Starting nearly two weeks later than they'd intended, the southern California sun is already blistering. Excited and nervous about their upcoming adventure, they set off into the wilderness.

HEAT EMERGENCIES

As they cross the Mojave Desert, Felicity notices her leg muscles keep cramping. Daytime temperatures have soared into the upper 90's, and the distances between water sources are long, so she's been conserving water, drinking rarely. But as the sun climbs higher and higher, she starts to feel tired deep in her bones. Every step is an effort, and her head is pounding. She's sweated through her shirt and is starting to feel nauseated. When they stop for lunch in the shade of a rock formation, she collapses to the ground and vomits. Finn hurries over and feels her forehead; she is cool and clammy to the touch.

HEAT EXHAUSTION

Heat exhaustion is characterized by extreme fatigue, headache, nausea and vomiting, dizziness, and profuse sweating. Your character's skin will be cool and clammy, their heart will race, and they'll be breathing fast. The lightheadedness and dizziness are caused by low blood pressure. Heat exhaustion is uncomfortable and unpleasant but is generally not life-threatening.

> *Seeing Felicity's state, Finn fills the rest of his canteen with Gatorade powder and makes Felicity drink it–slowly, so she doesn't vomit. They find a spot in the shade that has a breeze, and Felicity sits and sips until she's feeling better. They decide to wait there for a few hours until the heat of the day passes.*

Heat Exhaustion can be treated with electrolyte-rich fluids and finding whatever external method of cooling down is readily available, whether that is a shady spot or a cool bath. If your character doesn't improve within an hour, they should be taken to the hospital. There, Heat Exhaustion will be treated with IV fluids and external cooling, such as air conditioning and fans.

> *The next day, Felicity is feeling more like herself. She and Finn decide to start out before sunrise to avoid hiking during the heat of the day.*

HEAT STROKE

Heat Stroke, by comparison, is a life-threatening emergency. Common in the very old and the very young, Heat Stroke is differentiated from heat exhaustion by hyperthermia–a body temperature greater than 104°F. If your character is suffering from Heat Stroke, they will have hot, dry skin and may, paradoxically, be shivering. They may seem confused, tired, or delirious, and may have jerky or stilted movements. If untreated, Heat Stroke can lead to seizures and collapse of the cardiovascular system.

> While heat stroke victims generally don't sweat, it is possible for your character to sweat profusely and still have heat stroke, assuming they fit the other criteria. The uncertainty of the diagnosis–especially if your characters don't have a rectal thermometer handy–can add some serious tension. Remember; misdiagnosis can be fatal.

The first step in treatment for heat stroke is to bring down the victim's body temperature, fast. This includes cooling with water sprays, fans, ice packs in the groin and armpits, even cool IV fluids. Cold-water baths (and especially ice baths) are not recommended unless someone who knows what they're doing is monitoring the victim's rectal body temperature very closely. Cooling too fast can be just as dangerous as the heat stroke itself.

Victims of heat stroke need to be taken to a hospital, where they will be safely cooled, rehydrated, and stabilized. They'll also be given muscle relaxants, anti-seizure medications, and monitored closely for signs of organ dysfunction.

ALTITUDE EMERGENCIES

A few weeks into the hike, Finn and Felicity begin the ascent into the Sierra Nevada Mountain range. Today, their path leads upwards to Forester Pass, which at 13,200 feet is the highest point on the PCT. As they climb, Finn begins to feel dizzy and out of breath—well, more out of breath than he'd expect for wearing a 50lb backpack and climbing a trail so steep it feels more like a staircase than a path. Felicity, walking far ahead, doesn't seem to be having any trouble. His head is beginning to hurt as well, but he shakes it off—it's probably because he had so much trouble sleeping last night.

Altitude sickness happens–about 50% of people who climb to elevations higher than 8000 feet above sea level will experience it. Once you hit 10,000 feet, that number climbs to over 75%. Anyone can get it; your character can be fit as an Olympian and tough as nails, and they could still be brought low by this indiscriminate illness.

Altitude sickness, like most illnesses, has varying levels of severity. If your character has mild altitude sickness, they'll have a mild headache, feel a bit out of breath, and maybe a bit dizzy. They also might have some trouble sleeping, and not feel very hungry. Mild altitude sickness usually starts within a day of arriving at the high altitude, and your character will acclimate with time. If you want your character to avoid getting altitude sickness, have them hang out at high altitude (>8000 feet) for several days to acclimatize before they have to do anything crazy, like hike up a mountain. They can also take a medication called Acetazolamide as a prophylactic.

> Just because your character has acclimatized or is taking prophylaxis doesn't mean they can't get sick at higher altitudes. And not acclimatizing does not mean they will get sick. Altitude sickness is remarkably unpredictable.

By the time they reach the summit, Finn is having trouble catching his breath. His head pounds with the worst headache of his life, and his chest feels tight. Felicity, who's been waiting at the summit for him, hurries over and asks what's wrong, and why he's walking like he's drunk. Finn sits down on a rock, but he still can't quite catch his breath.

Moderate to severe altitude sickness is characterized by a severe headache, nausea and vomiting, fatigue, trouble breathing, and chest tightness. As long as your character stays at that altitude, these symptoms will continue to get worse. If your character becomes confused, can't breathe even though they've been resting, or can't walk, it's a sign that something is going very seriously wrong.

The two most serious types of altitude sickness are High-Altitude Pulmonary Edema (HAPE), also called Acute Mountain Sickness, and High-Altitude Cerebral Edema (HACE). Both occur because of fluid leaking out of your character's blood vessels due to the lower surrounding air pressure.

If your character has Acute Mountain Sickness (AMS) it means they have *Pulmonary Edema*–fluid filling their lungs and preventing them from getting oxygen into their bloodstream They'll have chest tightness, a cough that brings up thin whiteish fluid, and difficulty breathing, even when resting. Their lips, fingernails, and skin around their mouth will be tinged blue, and they'll be absolutely exhausted and weak. Untreated AMS leads to drowning–death due to fluid in the lungs–without your character being anywhere near a body of water.

> Pulmonary edema is not the same as "Dry Drowning," which occurs when a character dies of asphyxiation in a body of water, but has no liquid in their lungs due to a spasm of their airway.

HACE is due to *Cerebral Edema,* or fluid on the brain. Your character will have a severe headache, but they will also be confused and disoriented. They may have hallucinations or other psychotic behavior. Untreated HACE leads to coma and death.

Finn wants to take a nap at the top, but Felicity–alarmed by the blue-tinged skin around her brother's mouth, insists they need to go. Since it's early in the year, snow still covers the mountainside. Felicity, seeing the snow field, makes an immediate decision. Rather than follow the steep, rocky trail, she grabs her pack, then Finn's, and together they glissade down the snow field, dropping altitude as fast as possible. When they reach the treeline, Felicity grabs what she can out of Finn's pack–his raincoat, sleeping bag, and water bottle–and hands them to a still bewildered Finn. Then she shoulders her pack. and marches them downhill through the undergrowth until her altimeter reads 8000 feet above sea level. Only then does she allow them to make camp. Finn's headache has improved, and he's no longer feeling winded. He tells Felicity to rest while he makes camp—without his pack they no longer have a tent, but they still have sleeping bags and enough food to get them to town—if they can find it. They spend the rest of the evening planning how they will make it back to the trail without returning to the high elevations.

DROWNING

Drowning is defined as death due to suffocation after submersion in liquid. If your character didn't die, it was a near-drowning. Drowning is depressingly commonplace; more than 4,000 people die every year from drowning, most of them toddlers and teenage boys.[2]

The next morning, Finn and Felicity decide on a heading to take them back towards the trail. They've only been walking all day, making poor time through the thick underbrush, so it is late afternoon when they come to a river, still swollen with snowmelt. Debris rushes past, caught in the swift current. Felicity recognizes it as the river they were supposed to cross up near the pass—at a higher altitude where the water might have been shallower. They walk upstream until they find a shallow spot that looks safe to cross. Felicity is hesitant—the water is still moving fast, and she doesn't like the look of the occasional logs and branches floating past—but Finn insists that this is the fastest way back to the trail, and safety.

If your character is going to drown (or nearly drown), the first question to ask is why they drowned in the first place. Did they know how to swim? Was there a strong current that pulled them under? Were they under the influence of drugs or alcohol? Did they dive in and head their head at the bottom?

They cross carefully, using their trekking poles to stabilize themselves. The water is fast and icy cold, coming up to mid-thigh in places. They're halfway across when Felicity's foot slips on a rock and she falls backward, into the river. Icy water fills her mouth and nose as she tries to scream. The current has her in second, pulling her downstream throwing her against the rocks. She tries to slither out of her backpack, but it's caught between two rocks. She reaches down to unhook the belt-strap and escape, then something hard slams into the back of her head, and the world goes black.

Treatment of near-drownings is pretty straightforward: get the victim out of the water while protecting the C-spine, then evaluate the ABCs. If they're breathing on their own, they'll be given oxygen and taken to the hospital for fluids and monitoring. If they aren't breathing on their own, but have a pulse, your character will need to perform rescue breaths. Finally, if there is no pulse, your character will need to figure out how long the victim was submerged. If they were under for more than an hour, or if there are other clear signs of death (ie rotting, trauma, etc), the victim has drowned. If they were submerged for less than an hour, your character should start CPR.

Finn sees her go under, watches helplessly as she's carried downstream. He tries to grab her, but the current is too fast, and she's swept out of sight. He hurries to the far bank, then races downstream, screaming her name. Then he sees her floating face down in the water; by some miracle, her pack was caught between two boulders. It kept her in place, but also kept her underwater. He rushes in, unclips her from the pack—which is immediately caught by the current to float away—and drags her to the riverbank. She isn't breathing, but he can feel a pulse. Careful not to disturb her neck, he tilts her chin upwards and breathes twice into her open mouth. He does this twice more before she begins to cough, and he turns her onto her side just in time as she vomits up water.

State after Submersion	Action	Level of Care	Chance of Survival
Breathing Independently, no cough	None	Home	100%
Breathing Independently, +cough or trouble breathing	Give oxygen	Emergency Department	Very Good
Not Breathing, +pulse	Rescue Breaths	ICU	Good
Not Breathing, no pulse, <1 hour submerged	CPR	ICU	Slim
Not Breathing, no pulse, >1 hour	None	NA	Dead

Doing CPR on someone who was submerged for an hour may sound futile, but submersion in cold water helps preserve brain function. This preservation occurs for two reasons: first, the diving reflex–a primitive reflex initiated when the face is submerged in water–makes the heart beat slower and the victim hold their breath. This reflex decreases the water that gets into the lungs and also slows the body's metabolism. The cold temperature of the water also decreases metabolism and helps shunt blood towards vital organs. However, if you want the victim to emerge relatively unscathed–i.e., you don't want them to be totally brain-damaged–I'd keep the time of submersion to under 30 minutes.

COLD EMERGENCIES

Felicity sits up, rubbing the back of her head where the log hit her. She's grateful to be alive, but as the tops of the pine trees around them are tipped with gold, she realizes they are in a bad spot. The sun is setting, and they have no packs—no tent, no sleeping bags, no way to make fire. And she is soaking wet. Already, the temperature in the forest is dropping—Felicity remembers the last weather forecast she saw predicted lows in the '20s. Within minutes, she begins to shiver.

HYPOTHERMIA

Hypothermia occurs when your character's body is losing heat faster than it can make it, and the core body temperature drops to less than 95°F. Characters with mild hypothermia will shiver—once the hypothermia gets more severe, the shivering will stop. If your character is hypothermic, they'll exhibit slurred speech, clumsiness and loss of fine-motor coordination, confusion, forgetfulness, tiredness, and an unwillingness to do much of anything.

In moderate to severe hypothermia, your character will begin to get sleepy and delirious. They may even try to take off their clothes, a phenomenon called *paradoxical undressing*. As the hypothermia worsens, your character will become progressively less active and less awake, until they sink into a coma. Characters with severe hypothermia (body temperature less than 86°F) are at high risk of heart arrhythmias and pulmonary edema.

The first thing Felicity does is strip out of her wet clothes. Her fingers are so numb she has trouble pulling them off. She feels a little drunk—uncoordinated, nauseated, and a little silly—as Finn gives her his oversized rain jacket, and she huddles beneath it, shivering violently, while Finn goes in search of materials to start a fire—Felicity isn't sure if it's the cold, or the knock on the head she got earlier, but she's having trouble remembering things Finn told her. At his urging, she gets up and walks around their improvised campsite, rubbing her arms and shivering violently.

Hypothermia isn't just for sub-zero temperatures. Cold air, wind, and water can all contribute, as can your character's body size, age, and gender. Young children and the elderly are at particularly high risk of hypothermia.

While hypothermia can technically occur at any temperature less than body temperature, a good rule of thumb is that hypothermia is more likely to occur at any temperature lower than 50°F. If you add in additional factors–if it's a windy day, or if your character is wet, or if they're laying on a cold floor–that temperature increases. In 60-70°F water, hypothermia can occur within hours. Alcohol intoxication, dehydration, physical exhaustion, and certain medical conditions increase the risk of hypothermia.

> *Finn's years as an Eagle Scout, along with the backcountry training he and Felicity completed before starting their trek, finally comes in handy. He's able to get a fire started using his pocketknife and twigs, feeding it with dry wood from the forest floor. He even cobbles together enough pine boughs and ferns to make a shelter to keep off the wind. More ferns create a makeshift blanket, which he piles over Felicity, who is no longer shivering. Her skin is cold to the touch, and she keeps halfheartedly trying to pull off the jacket. Finn crawls in behind her, sandwiching her between the heat of the fire and the warmth of his body. He hopes it will be enough.*

Hypothermia is treated by rewarming–heated blankets, heat lamps, hot water bottles in the groin and armpits, warmed IV fluids, even inhaled warmed/humidified oxygen. At the hospital, they'll be monitored for signs of heart arrhythmias. Ventricular fibrillation–a deadly, pulseless heart rhythm–is particularly common.

> There's a saying in medicine about hypothermia:
>
> "No one is dead until they're warm and dead."

Most people recover well from hypothermia, providing they don't develop a deadly heart arrhythmia. If your character has severe hypothermia and no pulse, they can't be pronounced dead until they've been rewarmed.

FROSTBITE

> *Felicity spends the night in a muddled haze, fighting to stay awake. After the sun has risen and she can no longer see her breath puffing in the air, she peels off the layers of ferns and gets unsteadily to her feet–only to realize that her toes are white, hard, and completely numb.*

Frostbite happens when your character's skin and underlying structures are damaged by exposure to cold. Fingers, toes, ears, and cheeks are particularly sensitive. While exposed skin is particularly sensitive, frostbite can still occur under hats, jackets, and gloves. In sub-freezing temperatures, frostbite can occur in less than 30 minutes, but in extremely cold weather, if there is windchill, or if your character is wet, it can happen in minutes. There are three degrees of severity:

1. **Frostnip:** If your character has frostnip, their skin will be cold and red. They may feel pins and needles, or even numbness. If your character is properly warmed before frostnip progresses any further, they won't suffer any permanent damage. If not, they'll progress to…

2. **Superficial frostbite:** Superficial frostbite occurs when ice crystals form under the skin and deep tissue (call subcutaneous tissue). Skin damaged by superficial frostbite feels warm and swollen. At first, the skin might appear a deep red, but will quickly progress to white and frozen. After a day or two, the damaged skin will develop huge, fluid-filled blisters. As horrifying as these blisters look, they're actually a good sign; the blisters will pop and slough off, revealing healthy new skin underneath that is pink and very sensitive to touch.

3. **Deep frostbite:** Deep frostbite occurs when the cold injury penetrates down to the muscles, nerves, and bones. If your character has deep frostbite (also called third-degree frostbite), the tissue will initially appear blueish white and splotchy. It will feel numb, and the muscles beneath it won't work.

While Finn scavenges for more wood, Felicity warms her toes by the fire, careful not to let them get close enough to burn. At first, she can't feel the heat at all. Then, pain like fire shoots through her toes as the skin begins to thaw.

Frostbite is treated first with rewarming, placing the affected limb in a warm (not hot!) water bath. Pain control is very important during this stage, as rewarming can be exceedingly painful. Then the wound will need to be cared for. This may be as simple as wrapping it with sterile bandages to protect it from injury, or it may require removal of dead tissue (a procedure called debridement), or even amputation if necessary. Your character may also need antibiotics and a tetanus shot to prevent infection.

> Walking on frostbitten toes decreases the likelihood they'll be able to heal; your character should avoid walking on frostbitten toes if possible.

Without any supplies, Finn and Felicity decide their best chance is to find the trail and hope they run into other through-hikers with a satellite phone, as theirs was lost with Felicity's pack. Felicity's toes still hurt like h*ll, but without supplies, food, water, and shelter, saving her toes is the least of their worries.

> Do not rewarm a frostbitten area until your character is 100% sure it won't freeze again. Repetitive freezing/thawing inevitably leads to gangrene!

DEHYDRATION

Dehydration happens when your character is losing more water than they take in. It can occur due to insufficient fluid intake, too much fluid output (due to sweating, diarrhea, or vomiting), or a combination of the two.

> In cold temperatures, you can see water loss from the lungs, in the form of that white puff of condensation.

A normal, adult body loses water through sweat, breath, urine, and feces—even at rest in a room at a comfortable temperature, your character is losing water. If he doesn't drink enough to offset those fluid losses, he'll become dehydrated. Conversely, he can also become dehydrated if there's an increase in fluid output, such as profuse sweating, diarrhea, or vomiting.

After hiking all day through the subalpine forests of the Sierra Nevada mountains, Finn's mouth is dry and he feels exhausted. As they walk, he dreams of water, but without their water filtration system, or even the iodine tablets they kept as a backup, they can't drink safely from any of the streams. They take breaks, sitting in the shade, but whenever Finn stands up again, he feels dizzy, lightheaded, and can feel his pulse racing.

Thirst is the first sign of mild dehydration. As the dehydration becomes worse, your character will feel tired and parched, his mouth feeling dry as sandpaper. When he stands up, he'll feel a little dizzy and his heart will race—a phenomenon called *orthostatic hypotension*. He'll also pee less often, and when he does, his urine will become dark yellow and smelly.

If your character becomes severely dehydrated, he'll become incredibly fatigued. His brain will be foggy, and he'll have trouble thinking straight or making decisions. He will also have low blood pressure, even when lying down. When he presses down on his fingernails, they will stay pale, rather than refilling immediately with blood. He can also pinch his skin and it will stay upright, like eggs whites whipped into a merengue.

As night approaches, Finn realizes it has been over 24-hours since either he or Felicity has had even a sip of water. He's exhausted from hiking all day when they stop by a crystal-clear stream to make camp. Though he knows the risks—Giardia, Cryptosporidium, E. coli—he drinks the water anyway. Nothing has ever tasted so good.

STARVATION

Starvation occurs when your character ingests no food or other sources of calories for an extended period. Exactly how long your character can survive without food depends on many different variables, including their age, gender, body mass, and level of exertion. But the human body can survive a surprisingly long time without food—nearly two months if there's access to water[4]. Without water, that number drops anywhere from eight to twenty-one days.

> *As they walk through the thick understory, Felicity prays, thanking G-d that they didn't get sick from drinking the stream water. Her stomach rumbles so hard it feels like it's trying to eat itself. Luckily, she can see Mount Whitney through breaks in the trees and can navigate in the direction where the trail should be. She just prays they find it soon.*

While there's no way to exactly predict how your character will respond to starvation, there are general phases.

STAGES OF STARVATION

During the first few days of starvation, the body survives off complex carbohydrates stored in the liver and muscle. During this time, your character will feel tired, a little weak, and—of course—quite hungry, but they'll still mostly feel like themselves.

After about three days, the fuel stores in the liver will run out, and your character's energy needs will come mostly from their stored fat tissue, through a process called *ketosis*. During this stage, your character will lose a lot of weight. This stage of starvation is highly variable, as it is dependent on your character's fat reserves as well as their level of energy expenditure. However, once their Body Mass Index (BMI) drops below 13, they will have used up all their fat stores[5].

> A normal BMI is 19-25.

> *By the time they make camp for the third night off-trail, Felicity is exhausted. They've been bushwhacking for three days straight, with nothing to eat but a few handfuls of salmonberries. Luckily there are streams scattered throughout the forest, but they drink sparingly, and only from clear, fast-flowing water. Even with their precautions, Felicity feels as if she's in a waking dream; she's having trouble concentrating and has forgotten their heading on more than one occasion, causing them to spend hours backtracking.*

During this stage of starvation, your character will have extremely low energy and will find it difficult to concentrate. His testes will shrink, and he'll develop diarrhea, dry skin, and hair loss. He'll be very tired and will feel cold all the time. Paradoxically, he won't feel very hungry, and will also develop swelling in his feet and abdomen, making him look bloated.

After six days of wandering through the forest, Felicity is so exhausted she can barely walk. Their pace has slowed to a crawl, and it's everything she can do to force herself to put one foot in front of the other. She's developed diarrhea–whether from drinking the stream water or from hunger, she isn't sure–and she feels cold all the time, even during the heat of the day. The nights are torture, as she and Finn alternate tending the fire and cuddling together for warmth. She's so lost in her own muddled thoughts that she nearly walks right across the well-worn trail. When she realizes what it is, she falls to her knees in gratitude. They decide to make camp there; better to save their energy and wait for someone to come along.

Once your character's fat reserves have been used up, his body will start to break down lean proteins, particularly muscle. At first, this will mean a breakdown of skeletal muscles–the biceps, hamstrings, deltoids, and other large muscles that help move his body–but soon, the body will start breaking down heart muscle as well. It will also start breaking down other tissues–lung, ovaries, testis–anything to keep fueling the brain.

> Remember those pictures of starving African children with swollen bellies? That's **Kwashiorkor**, a subtype of starvation caused by a diet completely lacking in protein.

During this final stage of starvation, your character will start having significant neurologic symptoms, such as hallucinations and seizures. But he probably won't die of starvation; instead, he'll die from infections that his starving body can no longer fight off. If he somehow doesn't develop an infection, he'll eventually die of a heart attack or heart arrhythmia, as his body consumes heart muscle.

> Starvation due to severe calorie deficit is called **Marasmus**.

Felicity's prayers are answered, as another through-hiker walks past their camp just as the sun is dropping low over the horizon. He takes one look at the gaunt, exhausted siblings and uses his satellite phone to call for help. Within hours, Felicity and Finn are being helicoptered to the nearest hospital.

CHRONIC MALNUTRITION

Most cases of starvation in the US are not due to a sudden lack of calories. Instead, they're due to malnutrition–inadequate calories and nutrients. There are myriad causes of malnutrition, ranging from poor diet to malabsorption to eating disorders. Alcoholics and anorexics are notorious for having severe, prolonged nutritional deficiencies, and are at high risk of developing refeeding syndrome.

REFEEDING SYNDROME

In the hospital, Finn and Felicity are given IV fluids, a vitamin B shot, antibiotics, and an antiparasitic–for the infections they picked up from drinking untreated stream water–alongside a diet with a carefully calculated number of calories. They get blood drawn every meal, as the doctors closely monitor their electrolytes. Every day, the doctors increase their allotment of calories, and Finn realizes that he is starting to feel hungry again.

Reintroducing food to someone who has been starving or malnourished is a dangerous task. Food needs to be introduced slowly and deliberately, or else your character risks developing refeeding Syndrome, a potentially fatal imbalance of electrolytes, particularly phosphate.

If your character has refeeding syndrome, it will probably start around Day 4 of refeeding with general feelings of weakness, fatigue, and confusion. Those symptoms will then progress to heart failure and difficulty breathing. Their hands and feet will swell up, and they'll gain weight as their body retains fluids. They may start having seizures or heart arrhythmias. Untreated, refeeding syndrome can lead to coma and death.

Refeeding Syndrome is prevented by the slow, careful reintroduction of food and water, as well as close monitoring of blood electrolyte levels. If your character hasn't had anything to eat for at least ten days, or if he's lost more than 10% of his body weight in the last six months, expect for him to be hospitalized and put on a strict diet with daily blood tests monitoring his recovery[9].

BREAKING DOWN THE CLICHÉS:

HUMAN BITES

Baddi McBadass walks into the tavern, grabs the skinny blond man he's been tracking by the shoulders, then pops him one in the face. The man stumbles back against the bar, clutching his split upper lip. Baddi shakes the blood off his fist, pulls

> A young kid or elderly person with bite marks is a red flag for abuse.

a tooth from the knuckle of his scarred ring finger, then plops down onto the now-empty bar stool. As everyone stares, he pours the blond man's drink over the cuts on his knuckles, then orders another. On Blondie's tab, of course.

Not all human bites happen during combat. Kids bite, vampires bite, people who are intoxicated bite, the confused, the elderly, and the mentally disabled bite. But if a human bite does occur during combat, it's less likely to be the intentionally-sinking-their-teeth-into-your-character type of bite (an *occlusive bite*), and more of a punch to the teeth (*clenched fist, tooth-knuckle,* or *fight-bite injury*).

If your character punches someone in the mouth, they'll probably come away with a crescent of cuts along the first finger bones, between the knuckles of the hand and the first finger joint. These are called 'clenched fist injuries.' While they aren't as common as occlusive bites, if your character is a face-punching badass, they probably need to worry about it. That's because…

Human bites in film and television are *way* undertreated. After the protagonist gets bitten, they just put some gauze on the wound to stop the bleeding, then grimace and make some cocky joke about their challenger being sharper than they'd expected.

Turns out, that approach to human bites is likely to lead to some nasty complications. Human mouths are disgusting. At best, they're crawling with bacteria, including species of *Streptococcus* and *Staphylococcus* that are notorious for forming abscesses, damaging joints, infecting nearby bones, and worming their way into the bloodstream. At worst, they're carriers of life-threatening diseases, such as Hepatitis, Tetanus, and even Syphilis.

> There is no evidence that HIV can be transmitted through human bites.[10]

Human bites are treated similarly to cat bites–the wound is thoroughly washed, then left open (ie not stitched closed) to prevent the overgrowth of certain bacteria. If the bite involved a joint, it will be immobilized with a splint. If the bite was to the hand or scalp, they'll need X-rays to make sure no teeth fragments were left behind, and that there are no signs of bone infection. Then they'll get a tetanus shot and oral antibiotics. If there's any sign of bloodstream infection–fever, chills, or red streaks around the wound–or if your character probably won't be able to care for the wound, they'll be admitted.

> Bites to the penis are highly likely to get nasty infections.

KISS OF LIFE[6]

Sally McSwoony bravely pulls her crush from a lake but wait! He isn't breathing; time for some rescue breathing. As Sally's lips brush his, he wakes up–but enjoys having her lips on his so much that he pretends to still be unconscious for a few moments more. How romantic.

Rescue breathing is not sexy. Like I said before, human mouths are gross. Unless your character knows the drowning character super well, they are putting themselves at risk of getting a host of fun diseases, such as herpes, mononucleosis, and hepatitis, as well as the cold and flu. Add onto that some nasty morning breath, and mouth-to-mouth is a straight-up disgusting venture. Additionally, there's a strong likelihood the victim is going to vomit on your character—not just any old regurgitation, but projectile vomit straight to the mouth. This isn't just because they swallowed lake water; an improperly maintained airway can result in gastric insufflation. In other words, your character is breathing into their stomach, not their lungs. Eventually, the stomach gets too full and everything explodes out, reminiscent of those baking soda volcanoes we all made back in fourth grade. Just grosser.

Medical professionals never touch their lips to a patient's. They use a Bag Valve Mask (BVM), squeezing air into the victim's mouth. In their private lives, many medical professionals are grossed out enough by the idea of mouth-on-mouth that they carry one-way valve masks in their cars and purses so that if they ever have to do CPR in the field, they won't have to taste the other person.

Finally, if your character is doing rescue breathing, they should kneel to the side of the victim. Straddling them just makes it harder for the victim to breathe and for your character to make a good seal on the victim's mouth. And please have them check for breathing and a pulse before they start doing anything.

19. CONSCIOUSNESS & COMA

Gabriela is standing in the basement of the church's kitchen, rolling out tortillas for the evening's fundraiser and chatting with her best friend, Guadalupe. She's about to ask Lupe if she's enjoying having her house to herself—her two young sons are visiting their father in Mexico City for the summer—when Lupe cries out in pain. The rolling pin clatters to the ground as she clutches her head.

"What's wrong?" Gabriela asks, hurrying over. "Are you ok?"

Guadalupe just grimaces. "My...my head," she grits out. Then she sinks to the floor, pressing the heel of her hand tight against her right eye.

BACKGROUND

SOME OF THE MOST COMMON questions I'm asked are about comas. What is a medically induced coma? How long do they last? How does the character wake up? What injuries would require your character to be put into a medically induced coma?

First of all, "coma" isn't a diagnosis. It's a description of the character's level of consciousness; more specifically, it means that the character is not responding to any stimuli. The doctor could run around naked screaming her head off while playing the bongos on your character's testicles, and your character wouldn't so much as grimace. But consciousness is not an all-or-nothing state.

CONSCIOUSNESS

Consciousness ranges from fully awake and alert to completely unresponsive. It's a sliding scale, not a switch that you flip on and off. Your character isn't either awake, asleep, or in a coma; there's a lot of middle ground and most people in a hospital (especially an ICU) will end up falling

> **Oriented** means that your character knows who they are, where they are, why they're there, and the exact date. The medical abbreviation is **A&Ox4**

somewhere in the middle. Below are some levels of consciousness that could be used to describe your character.[1]

- **Alert and Oriented:** Awake and oriented to person, place, time, and purpose.
- **Alert:** Awake and responsive to the environment.
- **Clouded:** Inattentive, drifting in and out of sleep.
- **Confused:** Disoriented or bewildered.
- **Lethargic:** Drowsy, can only be woken up with loud voice or painful stimuli.
- **Obtunded** = Severely drowsy, never fully awake. Slow response to stimuli.
- **Stupor** = Sleeps all the time; only wakes to vigorous, painful stimuli, then falls right back to sleep.
- **Coma** = Unresponsive to any stimuli.

> **Painful stimuli** include sternal rubs, pinching the earlobe or the webs between fingers, or pressing something sharp against the nail bed.

Gabriela kneels on the ground beside her friend.

"Lupe! What's wrong?"

Guadalupe just vomits. Gabriela may just be a dermatologist, but she knows the signs of a burst aneurysm when she sees it. She grabs her phone from the pocket of her apron and calls 911. By the time the ambulance arrives, Guadalupe is fading in and out of sleep, waking only when Gabriella shakes her hard; even then, staying awake for only a few moments. Gabriela watches helplessly as the paramedics load her friend into the ambulance. Without asking permission, she jumps into the back, taking Lupe's hand in her own.

You may notice that these states of consciousness have a lot of overlap and aren't particularly precise, which is why medical professionals grade their patients' level of consciousness using the Glasgow Coma Scale.

GLASGOW COMA SCALE

The Glasgow Coma Scale (GCS) is used to evaluate your character's level of consciousness. Originally designed to be used after head trauma, it can also be used for other causes of coma and decreased consciousness, including stroke, toxic ingestions, and brain bleeds. The GCS has three components: eye-opening, verbal response, and motor response.

1. **Eye-opening** ranges from opening spontaneously (4 points) to not at all (1 point).

2. **Verbal response** ranges from speaking appropriately (5 points) to not making any noises (1 point).

3. **Motor response** ranges from obeying commands (6 points) to no movement (1 point).

A GCS of 3 is the lowest possible score. A GCS of 14-15 implies mild injury, while a score of 9-13 indicates more severe damage. A score of 3-8 indicates your character is in a coma.

COMA

At the ED, Guadalupe is surrounded by a team of doctors and nurses, starting IVs, drawing blood, and shining penlights into Lupe's eyes. Gabriela relays what happened, and Lupe is bustled off to the CT scanner. Then the ED doctor asks Gabriela about Guadalupe's family. Gabriela explains that Lupe's family still lives in Mexico, and the doctor asks if Gabriela would be willing to be Guadalupe's medical decision-maker. Gabriela agrees without question.

If your character is in a coma, their level of consciousness is so depressed that they cannot respond to any stimulus. There are lots of conditions that can cause a coma, ranging from drug or alcohol overdose to a traumatic brain injury. Some of these causes can be reversed with medications or surgery–if caught in time. Others may improve with time and still others are likely to be permanent. But any of these conditions can cause permanent brain damage or death if not caught and treated soon.

> Friends–even acquaintances–can be medical decision-makers if no one else is around, unless your character has already chosen a healthcare power of attorney.

Whether or not your character will make it out of their coma is determined by how severe and sustained the damage to the brain is. Blood, toxins, and imbalanced electrolytes can temporarily stun the brain, leading to a transient coma. But if the onslaught continues unabated, neurons–the brain cells that carry messages–start to die. And once that happens, the damage is irreversible.

Unlike many other cell types in the body, neurons cannot regrow. Once a neuron is dead, that brain function is lost. So, if you want your character to have a full, functional recovery after their coma, you better get them treatment fast.

When Guadalupe returns from the CT, Gabriela finds her even more drowsy than before. She tries to wake her friend, shaking her and calling her name, but Lupe only groans. A few minutes later, she doesn't move or respond at all, even when Gabriela pinches her earlobe hard. Gabriela calls for help, and Guadalupe is whisked away for emergency neurosurgery.

CAUSES

There are lots of conditions that can cause a coma; some are more reversible than others.

Potentially Reversible Causes

- Drug overdose (Ch. 17): alcohol, opioids, antidepressants, benzodiazepines, others.

- High Blood Pressure crisis (*Hypertensive Encephalopathy*).

- Diabetic Coma.

- Severe electrolyte imbalances.

- Vitamin Deficiencies: thiamine (B1), B12.

- Brain infections.

- Toxins: lead, ethylene glycol (antifreeze).

- Sustain*ed seizures (status* epilepticus).

Sometimes Reversible (or Partially Reversible) Causes

- Brain bleeds
- Brain Tumors
- Stroke
- Traumatic Brain Injury (TBI)

Rarely Reversible Causes

- Carbon Monoxide Poisoning.

- Severe lack of blood flow to the brain *(Anoxic/Hypoxic Brain Injury)*: caused by heart attack, drowning, or strangulation.

Of course, there will be exceptions–you've probably heard stories of someone whose family was told they would never wake up, who then woke up and walked out

> The radiology department (and CT scanner in particular) is notoriously dangerous. Critically ill or injured patients are sent to radiology for imaging without proper medical supervision, and promptly die. This shouldn't happen, obviously, but it does, and with enough frequency that the CT scanner earned its nickname: The Ring of Death.

> **Therapeutic hypothermia:** People are intentionally cooled after a massive cardiac arrest because low body temperature protects brain function. If your character nearly drowned, they'll have a much better chance of recovering if they'd been in a frozen lake than in a hot tub.

of the hospital. That *can* happen; our understanding of the brain is tenuous at best. But know that it is a rare exception. The general rule is that the earlier a condition is caught, the more likely it is to be reversible. Even the most reversible condition can be fatal if not treated promptly.

SEDATION

A few hours later, Guadalupe is brought to her room in the ICU. Gabriela's throat tightens as she sees her friend—her head shaved and covered in bandages, drains and tubes peeking out from beneath her hospital gown. The doctors tell Gabriela that Guadalupe burst a berry aneurysm—a bulging blood vessel in her brain that burst. It was the blood that caused her sudden, horrible headache, and the increasing pressure on her brain that caused her to lose consciousness. Gabriela nods—she knows all this, but she lets the young doctor explain anyway. They were able to stop the bleeding in time to prevent the brain from herniating, but there was a lot of blood on her brain. They won't know the full extent of her injuries—or her ability to heal from them—for a while. In the meantime, she'll be sedated for pain control—and so she doesn't pull out her tubes—but the doctors are cautiously optimistic that she will make a good recovery.

> **Brain herniation** occurs when elevated pressures inside the skull force the skull down through the hole leading to the spinal cord.

DEFINING SEDATION

Sedation is the use of medications to artificially depress a person's consciousness. Done properly, sedation results in a decreased level of consciousness, rather than complete unresponsiveness.

Sedation is used in many different circumstances, from pain control to behavioral regulation. Anyone who's ever had surgery, or even had a tooth pulled, has experienced sedation. If your character is in severe pain—fractures requiring traction, severe burns, multiple wounds—they may need to be sedated. Ventilated patients often need to be sedated as well.

> **Snowed** is slang for heavily sedated.

Anesthesiologists and critical care specialists use sedation protocols to give your character the lowest level of sedation needed. Oversedation can be extremely dangerous, responsible for everything from decreased quality of sleep to increased mortality. For that reason, doctors will monitor your sedated character very closely.

RECOVERY

Recovering from sedation is usually pretty quick and easy–on the scale of minutes to hours. Your character will march up the sliding scale of consciousness until they're awake and alert. How long this process takes is entirely dependent on the medication and dose they were given, though your character may feel groggy for hours after sedation.

SEDATED DOES NOT MEAN COMATOSE

Remember, if your character is sedated, they'll be at least minimally responsive to their environment. They may open and close their eyes, murmur incoherently, or squeeze a loved one's hand. This means they are *not* in a coma. However, there are a few rare instances when your character might need to be sedated so deeply that they become comatose.

> Actually, there's a third reason: surgery. If you've ever been put under general anesthesia, congrats! You've survived a medically induced coma.

THERAPEUTIC COMA (BARBITURATE COMA, MEDICALLY INDUCED COMA)

There are two reasons your character would intentionally be so deeply sedated that they are completely nonresponsive: severe brain injury or status epilepticus. For both, the barbiturate coma is a dangerous last resort, used only when doctors have run out of other options.

On the second day in the ICU stay, the pressure inside Guadalupe's brain begins to rise. The doctors say it is the brain's reaction to all the blood. They try everything to stop it; checking to make sure her drain is working, putting the head of her bed at a 45-degree angle, giving medications and concentrated fluids to try and pull the fluid out of her brain tissue, but nothing works. Even though she's breathing on her own, they intubate her and put her on a ventilator so that they can control her breathing. Finally, the doctors tell Gabriela that they need to put Lupe into a therapeutic coma to decrease the activity of her brain and help the swelling go down. Gabriela is told to wait in the ICU's waiting room. When she returns, Guadalupe has been intubated and hooked up to the ventilator, her shaved head now covered in EEG wires. Gabriela stands beside her friend, taking her hand, but Lupe doesn't respond. The only sounds are the whooshing of the ventilator and the beeping of instruments.

> **Electroencephalograms** (EEGs) monitor the electrical activity of the brain.

BRAIN INJURY

If your character has had a significant brain injury, such as a severe TBI or a massive stroke, a therapeutic coma may be used to help control the brain swelling. And I'm talking about *severe* injuries, where the CT brain is so bloody it looks like something out of Resident Evil. The basic idea is that, like anywhere else in your body, the tissue's response to injury is to swell up as it tries to recover. Only, the brain is stuck in the hard, immobile casing of the skull. Too much brain swelling leads to an increased intracranial pressure (ICP) which leads to herniation–the brain squishing out of the hole leading down into the spine–which leads to death. So, doctors do everything in their power to get swelling to go down, ranging from surgery to open up the skull or drain the fluid, to repositioning the head of the bed. But one of the most important things doctors can do is to quiet the brain.

Brain activity leads to increased ICP. So, doctors give sedating medications–barbiturates like pentobarbital or propofol–to quiet the brain, placing them in a coma. If your character is in a barbiturate coma due to brain injury, they will be unresponsive and dependent on a ventilator for *at least* 72 hours. During that time, they will receive round-the-clock care from the intensive care team, and a neurologist will carefully monitor the recovery of their brain function.

REFRACTORY STATUS EPILEPTICUS

Status epilepticus is an unrelenting seizure, defined as a seizure that lasts for more than five minutes. It is a life-threatening medical emergency. If the seizure doesn't respond to treatment and continues beyond five minutes, it is considered refractory.

Refractory status epilepticus (RSE) is stopped in much the same way you'd stop a gasoline fire–by smothering it. High-dose barbiturates (usually pentobarbital) are given by IV, smothering the electrical activity of the brain and putting your character into a therapeutic coma.

COMA MONITORING

While your character is in a coma–medically induced or not–they will be closely monitored by a team of healthcare professionals. Intensive care specialists will monitor their blood pressure, electrolyte levels, and vital signs, among other things. Every day, neurosurgeons will monitor drains, surgical sites, and intracranial pressures while neurologists perform intensive neurologic exams. The neurologists will also monitor brain function through a series of EEGs. EEGs are time-consuming–a technician has to place 25 electrodes in a specific pattern all over the skull–bulky, and finicky, so most coma patients will receive only one or two EEGs. But if your character is in a therapeutic coma, they will receive constant EEG monitoring.

Gabriela returns to the ICU early the next morning. To her surprise, there's a doctor already at Guadalupe's side. Gabriela watches with interest as the doctor shines a light into Lupe's eyes, then moves her head back and forth. He calls Guadalupe's name, then rubs his knuckles hard against her breastbone. Then he moves to one side and starts tapping a double-sided, silver reflex hammer against her arms and legs, flexing and extending each joint. Finally, he sharply flexes Lupe's bare feet, running the sharp point of the reflex hammer along the sole. Gabriela frowns as Guadalupe's toes splay outward; she knows the Babinski reflex is a sign of brain damage.

The neurologic exam is a hands-on evaluation of your character; the doctors won't just listen to your character's heart and lungs and peace out. It's a thorough examination, but it doesn't necessarily have to take forever—a neurologist in a hurry can do the full exam in less than two minutes. But if you're writing a character in a coma, please have a doctor come into the room that does more than just listen to their heart.

RECOVERY

If your character is in a therapeutic coma due to brain injury, they'll need to stay in the coma for a minimum of 72 hours. Then, once the intracranial pressure has normalized, and has stayed normal for 48 hours, your character can be weaned off the barbiturates.[3] If they were put in the therapeutic coma due to Refractory Status Epilepticus (RSE), they'll start being weaned off 24 hours after the electrical storm of seizure activity has calmed down.[4]

The first step to recovery from a medically induced coma is to stop the barbiturates depressing their brain function. After that, they're just like any other coma patient; the extent of the damage to their brain will determine the course of their recovery.

> Note that the length of a medically induced coma is measured in hours.

One week later, Guadalupe's brain pressures have stabilized. She's weaned off the barbiturates, then the ventilator. She is breathing on her own, but she doesn't wake up, just lays there with her eyes closed even when Gabriela calls her name or pinches her earlobe. When Gabriela asks when she'll wake up, the doctors shake their heads—she had significant brain damage. Only time will tell.

Recovery after a coma depends entirely on why your character was in the coma in the first place. Coma due to opioid overdose can be reversed in minutes with a single dose of Naloxone, while recovery from a coma due to a brain bleed may take days, weeks, or even months as the blood is reabsorbed, and new blood flow returns to the tissue.

Returning to consciousness is a slow process–your character will gradually work their way up the levels of consciousness. They may begin to move at the sound of the doctor's voice, open their eyes upon command, or mumble incoherently. Most of the time, this process happens over days or weeks. Most comas last for less than four weeks; the longer the coma lasts, the less likely your character is to recover.[8]

OUTCOMES

Outcomes for comas vary as widely as the potential causes, and it can be very hard to predict who will recover and who will not. Generally, infection and metabolic causes–such as drugs, blood sugar, toxins, and electrolyte imbalances–have the best prognosis. Brain bleeds and strokes tend to have the worst outcomes, with a survival rate of less than 5%.[7] Conditions causing low blood flow to the brain, such as drownings, strangulations, severe hemorrhage, and heart attacks, have the highest rate of a persistent vegetative state.[7]

If your character was put in a therapeutic coma, chances are their outlook for recovery is going to be poor.

Somewhere between 40-60% of people with Refractory Status Epilepticus die because of it.[5] If they do survive, they are likely to be left with severe disability; one study found that every patient admitted for RSE had complications in the hospital, and 75% had a severe decline in their mental functioning after recovery.[6]

Recovery from a therapeutic coma after brain injury is similarly grim. Only about 20% of people with GCS of 3-5 will survive, and less than half of those will achieve a life with only mild-to-moderate disability.[2] This means that, even if your character is lucky enough to be in the 5-10% of coma patients who experience a "good recovery," they still may have disabilities severe enough that they can no longer work.

> *Gabriela returns the next weekend to check on Guadalupe. She's no longer in the ICU, but other than that, not much has changed; Lupe still doesn't open her eyes or say words, though one arm sometimes moves aimlessly on the bed. The doctors say that Lupe will need to transfer to a skilled nursing facility soon. Gabriela is shocked–Guadalupe still looks so sick. But her body is doing well, and she doesn't need further medical treatment besides nursing care. A social worker helps Gabriela pick out a facility, and Lupe is transferred there the next day.*

PERSISTENT VEGETATIVE STATE (PVS)

Not everyone who survives a coma will return to full consciousness. Your character's body may recover from their accident or illness, but not their brain. They'll be able to breathe on their own, maintain their heart rate, blood pressure, body temperature, and other functions, but they'll have no self-awareness or ability to interact with their environment–including people. This condition is called a vegetative state, and it occurs when the brain was so drastically and irreversibly injured that only the lowest, most basic level of functioning exists. If it lasts more than 1 month, it's a persistent vegetative state.[9]

> *One month later, Gabriela visits Guadalupe in her new home—a double room in a nursing facility that smells of pine sol and old person. Lupe lays on a hospital bed, eyes open, one half of her body completely immobile, the other occasionally twitching or jerking. Her eyes rove ceaselessly from left to right, never lingering on anything. Gabriela claps her hands in front of her friend's face, but Lupe doesn't blink, doesn't stop that ceaseless movement of her eyes. Occasionally, she makes a soft grunting sound. Gabriela takes her hand and feels her friend's fingers close around hers. She wants to believe it's Lupe, wants to believe she's doing this on purpose—but she knows it isn't. The palmar grasp reflex is a primitive reflex, normal in babies, but a sign of brain damage in adults. Instead, she turns on her phone and starts up Lupe's favorite reggaeton album, then pulls up photos of Lupe's sons and starts showing them to her one at a time. But Lupe's eyes don't so much as linger over the photographs. Gabriela leaves an hour later, wondering if her time would have been better spent talking to a rock.*

> PVS functionality isn't too different from a newborn, whose higher brain hasn't kicked in yet. Newborns can grasp, suckle, and look around, but they don't have the brainpower to do it on purpose...yet.

A vegetative state is confusing and heartbreaking, because your character will look awake, but will be totally unresponsive to their environment. Someone in a vegetative state can:

- Have sleep-wake cycles
- Yawn, chew, swallow, even grunt.
- Make facial movements that can approximate a smile or a frown
- Tear up.

- Move their limbs, even grasp objects placed in their hand.
- Move their eyes as if looking around.

But these are all basic reflexes. They can't react to external stimuli, can't move or speak intentionally. They can't even make eye contact. Though our grasp of consciousness is far from complete, as far as science has been able to determine, those in a vegetative state have absolutely no evidence of consciousness.

The prognosis for someone in a vegetative state is dismal; most people die within six months. Less than 25% live beyond five years. However, as you've probably seen on daytime television, someone in a persistent vegetative state *can* develop consciousness months, even years after the inciting incident. But don't get your hopes up.

About 3% of people in a vegetative state will go on to develop some form of consciousness.[10] It's most likely during the first six months–a year if the coma was caused by a traumatic brain injury. After that, the likelihood drops practically to zero. But for the vast majority of people, improvement does not mean walking out of the hospital. Many will simply make the slight upgrade to a minimally conscious state. Few will ever live independently again; none will go back to the level of functioning they had before the incident.

> A **minimally conscious state** is a small step up from a vegetative state. People can make eye contact, purposefully grasp objects, and echo–answer a one-word question with the same word. It isn't much, but it's evidence of consciousness.

BREAKING DOWN THE CLICHÉS:

MEDICALLY INDUCED COMA

> *He was jumped in a dark parking lot, beaten to an inch of his life. They broke his legs and his ribs, shattered his spleen, and severed his spinal cord. The ambulance got there just in time—he was taken to the hospital and, after surgery, put into a medically induced coma to heal.*

People aren't put into comas to heal–they are sedated. Maybe it's just semantics, but we're writers; we need to be careful with language. Someone who is sedated and put on a ventilator has a *much* better chance at survival and recovery than someone with a major brain bleed who was put into a therapeutic coma to keep their swelling brain from squelching out of the hole in their skull.

THE AWAKENING

> *He's been in a coma for twelve years; the doctors say there's almost no brain function left. His children have grown up and moved on, but his wife hasn't given up hope. She still visits him every day, holding his hand as she watches him sleep. But one day, his eyes blink open. He looks lovingly into her eyes, brow furrowed. "Where am I?"*

Nope. Nope. Nope. I'm sorry, but it doesn't happen that way. "Awakenings"–the media term for someone returning to consciousness after a persistent vegetative state–*can* happen, though it's rare. But people don't go straight from comatose to fully conscious in the blink of an eye. And they *will* have significant, residual disability. If you don't believe me, read the Wikipedia page on people who've awoken from a coma.[11] It's a short list.

REAL TALK

I'm hammering on this point because it broke my heart how families would cling to the thought of their loved one "waking up" from their coma. They'd seen enough soap operas or Hallmark movies to hold out hope that their loved one would just snap out of it one day. Unfortunately, the chances of that happening are worse than winning the lottery.

Yet so many people truly believe that their loved one will wake up as their old self. And while this phenomenon may have more to do with the human tendency to cling to shreds of hope, no matter how thin, decades of tired plot twists revolving around comas certainly hasn't helped. As writers, we need to do better.

20. VENTILATORS

Hanami's had a fever for almost a week now, along with a wracking cough and chills so severe her whole body shakes. She had a positive COVID test a few days ago and was told to stay home and quarantine, but her husband drove her to the ER when she started having trouble breathing.

Now, that difficulty breathing is getting worse. Every breath is a struggle, and she's starting to feel lightheaded. She presses the call button for the nurse, who immediately goes to get the doctor. By the time the doctor arrives, Hanami is leaning forward, hands on her knees as she gasps for air. The doctor listens to her lungs, then explains that she is desaturating—her oxygen levels are plummeting despite her increased breathing rate and the mask blowing oxygen into her face. She needs to be intubated and placed on a ventilator.

BACKGROUND

A MECHANICAL VENTILATOR IS A COMPLICATED instrument that gives breaths at a designated volume, oxygenation, humidity, and rate. Characters who need a ventilator are not getting enough oxygen into their blood, either because they aren't breathing at all, aren't breathing sufficiently, or are working too hard to breathe. If the problem isn't with their breathing—say, their heart isn't beating, or a clot is blocking blood flow to the lungs—ventilating isn't going to do much good on its own.

> If your character needs CPR, they may be intubated and given breaths with a Bag Valve Mask (BVM), but they will not be hooked up to a ventilator unless their heart starts to beat again.

THE PROCESS

After explaining the process of intubation and ventilation to Hanami, the doctor asks for her consent. Hanami is so out of breath she can't force out the single syllable, so she just nods. Then she lies back on the table, holding her husband's hand as she watches the nurse inject a medication into the IV in her arm.

A WRITER'S GUIDE TO MEDICINE

INTUBATION

Intubation involves using a laryngoscope—a stainless steel tool inserted into the back of the throat—to help open the airway so the doctor can guide a flexible plastic tube, called an *Endotracheal tube* (ET tube) down through the trachea and into the large airways of the lungs.

Intubation is an uncomfortable procedure. If your character doesn't have a pulse or isn't breathing at all, they'll be intubated without delay. However, if they're still conscious, they'll usually be given sedating medications (and possibly a paralytic) to make the procedure easier.[1]

VENTILATION

Once intubated and hooked up to the ventilator, your character will be lightly sedated, meaning sedated only to the point where they are calm and comfortable—somewhere between awake and alert, and drowsy but responding to commands. They are *not* in a medically induced coma (Ch. 19). This means that your character can be awake and alert while ventilated and may even be able to communicate by writing notes.

THE EXPERIENCE

Hanami is woken by a scratchy feeling at the back of her throat. She's laying on her stomach in a hospital bed. Out of the corner of her eye, she can see a white machine with a bunch of dials and plastic tubing that connects from the machine to her mouth. There's a whooshing sound, and she feels air pushed into her lungs. She tries to fight it but her chest expands, then deflates against her will. She reaches up to touch her face—there's a tube in her mouth, locked in place with a plastic stabilizer and tape stuck all over her face and neck. Panic rises inside her, and she starts to pull at the tubes, ignoring the screaming of alarms from the machine beside her bed. A nurse rushes in, telling her to stop, and injects something into her IV.

> Ventilated patients with COVID are "proned," meaning laid on their stomach to improve the ventilation to their lungs.

Being ventilated is *not* a pleasant experience. Your character will be able to feel the ET tube in their throat—a constant scratching they can do nothing about. They'll have tape sticking to their face and a mess of wires and IV tubes required stuck all over them. They

> **Bucking the vent** is slang for the patient trying to breathe at their own pace, rather than with the ventilator. It can be painful to watch.

won't be paralyzed, but the sheer volume of equipment attached to them will make it difficult to move much more than their hands.

If your character can initiate breaths on their own, the ventilator might just assist the breathing. But if the ventilator is set to breathe at a fixed rate, your character won't be able to breathe at their natural rate. This disunion can lead to intense feelings of suffocation and panic, even though labs show their blood is getting enough oxygen. The experience of being ventilated is so traumatizing that a recent study found that more than 30% of people who'd been ventilated in the ICU had PTSD from the experience.[2]

> *Hanami's world becomes a confusing whirlwind of pain and panic. She fades in and out of sleep; every time she wakes, she can feel the tube in her throat, the air forcing its way into her lungs. Her mouth feels dry as sandpaper. Sometimes, it feels like she's breathing too fast, other times, too slow. She wishes she could just sleep, but she's too uncomfortable, and something is always beeping. Sometimes her husband is there beside her, sometimes he isn't. Hanami feels as if she's trapped in a nightmare.*

Ventilators are also loud. Every breath is a soft whoosh and a click. They have an incredible variety of different beeps and alarms—one doctor told me she kept track of them by their little melodies, assigning them lyrics like "Not a big deal" and "Holy sh*t" and "Dead. Dead. Dead."[9] Because of the overabundance of alarms, doctors and nurses eventually start tuning them out. But leaving alarms to beep—even the benign ones—can be a source of significant anxiety to your character, who probably doesn't know that those terrifying beeps aren't signaling something serious. At the very least, your character will be cranky after being kept awake all night by the d*mn alarms.

> Alarm fatigue is real, especially in the ICU. There are so many different things beeping that nurses and doctors stop noticing them. For your character, all the beeping can be a source of significant anxiety and frustration.

WEANING OFF THE VENTILATOR (VENT WEANING)

> *One day, Hanami wakes to see her nurse standing over her, watching her carefully. Hanami waits for the ventilator to force air into her lungs, but it doesn't come. She breathes in, hesitant at first, then more confidently. It feels so good to breathe on her own, even if it is through the tube. The nurse smiles, then tells her she's passed her breathing trial. He hooks Hanami up to the ventilator again, telling her it's only temporary until the doctor can come in and extubate her. Hanami can't wait—every breath feels like a violation.*

Finally, the doctor comes in and pulls the tube from Hanami's throat. Hanami sputters and coughs, relieved her ordeal is finally over.

Being on a ventilator will put your character at risk for a host of new issues, including ventilator-associated pneumonia. For that reason, doctors try to get their patients off the vent as soon as possible. There are three steps to getting your character off the vent.[3]

Readiness testing: Ensure your character is medically stable and that whatever condition put them on the vent has resolved.

1. **Spontaneous Breathing Trial (SBT)**: Someone (usually the nurse) turns off the pressure support on the ventilator to see if your character breathes on their own.

> Your character does not need to be fully awake in order to be extubated. They only need to be awake and responsive enough able to follow simple commands.[4]

   No = Back on the vent

   Yes, but they're struggling, or their blood oxygen levels drop = Back on the vent

   Yes, and they maintained their blood oxygen levels = Extubate

If your character fails their SBT, don't worry! They can always redo it the next day.

> SBTs are repeated daily until your character passes, or they hit the three-week mark.

2. **Extubation:** The doctor or Respiratory Therapist (RT) removes the ET tube, so your character is once again breathing on their own. Then they're given oxygen and monitored closely in the ICU for 12-24 hours.

But what if your character is not able to be weaned off the ventilator?

TRACHEOSTOMY

There are lots of reasons your character might not be able to be weaned off the ventilator. Their underlying condition might not have resolved, they might have developed complications, or they might just be too sick. Unfortunately for them, when it comes to mechanical ventilation through an ET tube, there's a deadline.

3 weeks.

This number can fluctuate a bit, but for the most part, if your character hasn't been able to wean off the ventilator after three weeks, they are considered to need persistent mechanical ventilation (PMV). And at that point, your character (or their family) is going to have some tough choices to make.

Intubation is not a long-term solution. The longer that tube is down their throat, the higher the likelihood of life-threatening complications like pneumonia, ulcers, and tears in the lining of the esophagus.[5] After three weeks, the risk-benefit balance starts to shift, and continued ET tube placement becomes more dangerous than beneficial.

So, what do people needing prolonged ventilation do?

The answer is that they get surgery to permanently open a passage to their airways, called a tracheostomy. It's a surgical opening in the neck, just below the vocal cords. A short tube is inserted into this hole, and secured in the neck, providing stable, secure access to the windpipe. That tube is then connected to the ventilator.

A tracheostomy isn't without danger–it can bleed or get infected just like an ET tube–but it is much safer and more stable. It can also be reversed if your character improves.[7] However, it requires a surgical procedure, with all its attendant risks. For some, the risk of a tracheostomy outweighs its benefits.

REAL TALK: CHOOSING A TRACHEOSTOMY

For many families, the decision to proceed to a tracheostomy is representative of a much bigger choice: pursue aggressive medical treatment or let their loved one die.

It's an incredibly difficult decision. Choosing a tracheostomy means that your character will live–but at what cost? Life on a ventilator–even with a tracheostomy–is exceedingly uncomfortable. What sort of quality of life will your character have? What

> Most of the time, this choice is made by the loved ones on behalf of an unconscious character. But sometimes, a character is conscious and must decide themselves: die today or risk a future of suffering and becoming a burden.

sort of financial and emotional burden will this place on their family? Can family members dedicate their lives to caring for your character, or afford 24-7 nursing care? If your character is extremely ill, has major brain damage, or has a terminal illness, is a tracheostomy just prolonging the inevitable?

On the other hand, choosing not to proceed with the tracheostomy means that your character will be extubated, and die. Death could come in minutes or days, but it will come. Choosing not to perform a tracheostomy means choosing death.

Now, it's important to note that doctors

> Hospice is almost always free. Ventilator care, on the other hand, is incredibly expensive. Like it or not, cost often becomes a factor when making this decision.

don't just yank out the tube and let your character suffocate to death. If your character chooses not to proceed with the tracheostomy, they'll be referred to a palliative care team (Ch. 7) who will prescribe medications and therapies designed to keep your character comfortable. Throughout the process, the hospice team will provide support for the family and loved ones and will do everything in their power to make your character's transition to death as seamless and painless as possible. But your character *will* die.

Choosing whether to pursue tracheostomy may be the single most difficult choice in medicine. It has long-term financial, emotional, social, and moral repercussions. While families often make the decision together, in the end, there is always a single decision-maker (usually the spouse or your character's Power of Attorney) who gets the final word. What happens if loved ones disagree? If the decision-maker is at odds with the rest of the family? If one character makes a decision that creates an untenable financial and/or social burden for others?

> One study found that the cost of home mechanical ventilation was $7,050/month. Care in a facility jumped to $21,570/month. These costs are usually not covered by insurance.[8]

It can tear a family apart.

BREAKING DOWN A CLICHÉ: VENTILATOR = COMA

Sarah Sadsack sits beside her husband, holding his hand. Unable to breathe due to pneumonia, he's been in a medically induced coma for weeks. But each time she squeezes his hand, he squeezes right back, as if to let her know he's thinking of her too.

Sarah's husband isn't in a coma; he's sedated. And sedating a character is not the same thing as putting them in a medically induced coma.

If your character is ventilated, they'll be sedated with medications to keep them comfortable. Their level of consciousness should range anywhere from awake and relaxed (yes, your character can be *awake* while on a ventilator), to asleep but arousable. This means that they can squeeze your character's hand when instructed to or might open their eyes to the sound of their name.

If your character is in a coma, they won't respond to anything, even pain. A coma has a terrible prognosis—most people who've survived a coma will have months of recovery ahead of them, as well as residual brain damage. On the other hand, most people who are sedated and put on a ventilator can expect to return to their daily lives once they've healed from whatever illness or injury that put them on the vent in the first place. There's a big difference. Don't get it wrong.

21. DEATH & DYING

Iva settles onto the chair beside her father's bed. He's sleeping—it seems like he's always sleeping these days—but his breathing is louder than yesterday, more gurgly. The hospice nurse steps into the room, and Iva moves aside to let her work.

"His blood pressure is good," the nurse says, her voice low and respectful. "He can always request more pain medications if he needs them."

Iva nods, her throat tight. Her father's cancer has spread everywhere—his bones, his liver, even his brain—and he always seems to be in pain. She wonders if that's why he sleeps so much.

DEATH OCCURS WHEN THE BODY'S crucial functions are irreversibly damaged to the point where the body ceases to operate.[1] The most common causes of adult deaths in the US are heart disease, cancer, and accidents (in that order), but you certainly aren't limited to those. Death can look very different in different people. Your character can be old, young, healthy, or ill. They may wait to die until a beloved family member has said goodbye, or it may happen in the rare moment while they're alone. If you're writing a death scene, you have the license to get creative.

> A **hospice house** is a comfortable healthcare facility where your character may choose to spend the end of their life (See Ch. 7).

SIGNS & SYMPTOMS

Death can happen quickly and unexpectedly. But if your character has a chronic, terminal disease, there are certain signs you can add into your writing that will signal they're about to kick the bucket. Their appetite decreases, they sleep more, and they'll poop and pee less frequently. Because they have less energy, they'll be less able to hold conversations or interact with their loved ones.

As death approaches, they'll get weaker. They may be unable to lift a spoon to their mouth or pull up the blankets when they're cold. And they *will* get cold, their body temperature decreasing, especially in the extremities, which may turn purplish-blue or mottled. Other vital signs, such as blood pressure and heart rate, will drop as well.

> *As Iva is about to head home, her father stirs.*
>
> *"Iva?" he croaks.*
>
> *"Yes, Abba?" Iva asks, hurrying to his side.*
>
> *"What time is it? Where am I?"*
>
> *"We're at the hospice house, dad. And it's almost dinner time. Are you hungry?"*
>
> *He hasn't eaten in days. Her father looks down at the pile of blankets covering him, a gnarled finger tracing the seam of the wedding quilt Mom sewed for them years ago.*
>
> *"You said dinner time? Any chance there's chocolate cake?"*
>
> *Iva stifles a watery laugh. "I bet I can find you some. Hold on."*
>
> *She's reluctant to leave her dad, even for a second, but he hasn't been lucid enough to ask for anything in weeks. She hurries into the hallway, finds the nurse, and relays the request. Iva returns to her Abba, who's sitting up in his bed. A few minutes later, the nurse returns with chocolate cake and Iva and Abba spend the next hour eating and talking like they used to before he got sick. Then, as suddenly as it came, the energy drains out of him.*
>
> *"I'm tired, Iva," he says, his voice thin and brittle once more. "You should go home. I'll talk to you tomorrow."*

One sign that your character is about to die is, paradoxically, a sudden improvement. Known as *terminal lucidity*, your dying character may suddenly regain their energy, become interested in food and water, and seem more lucid than they have in a long while. They may become restless or seem at peace. This sudden peak in energy, colloquially called the "end-of-life rally," is a well-described phenomenon that is a hallmark of impending death. It may last for days or only a few minutes. Either way, it is temporary, and a sign that your character will soon be dead. How would your protagonist react to having their hopes raised and then dashed in such a spectacular manner?

> *When Iva returns the next morning–bearing another piece of chocolate cake– she's met by the nurse from yesterday. But when she tries to thank her for finding the cake, the nurse just shakes her head.*

"I'm sorry, dear," she says, "your father isn't responding anymore. I don't think he has much time left."

Heart in her throat, Iva hurries up to Abba's bedside. He's asleep, though sometimes he lets out a low, horrible moan. His breaths are loud and wet—Iva uses the suction nozzle at the side of his bed to suck out the thick, goopy mucus from the back of his throat.

Towards the end, your character may hallucinate or become confused. They may seem in pain, moaning and groaning, or muttering incoherently. As they become weaker, they'll slip out of consciousness. Unable to protect their airway, mucus and saliva accumulate in the back of their throat, causing a gurgling noise known as the "Death Rattle." This labored breathing can last anywhere from a few hours to a few days, but it is almost universally a sign that the end is near.

> The death rattle can last for days and is treated by suctioning out the secretions.

TYPES OF DEATH

There are two types of death: cardiopulmonary and brain death.

CARDIOPULMONARY DEATH

As Iva watches, her father's breaths come further and further apart. She finds herself counting the seconds in between, wondering each time if this breath is his last. Finally, there are no more breaths.

Cardiopulmonary death is what most people think of when they think of death. The heart has stopped, and your character is no longer breathing. It is an irreversible cessation of the cardiac and pulmonary functions necessary for life.

The key word here is irreversible. If someone's heart stops and they don't have a DNR, your character should start CPR immediately because there is a chance that whatever just happened is reversible. ACLS uses medications to try and reverse the damage and get the heart beating again. Sometimes it works. But only sometimes.

> See Ch. 15 for more on CPR and ACLS.

If someone starts CPR, but the victim doesn't regain a heartbeat, the doctor running the Code eventually has to decide when to stop lifesaving measures and call the time of death. And it is *incredibly* arbitrary. There are almost no guidelines for when to throw in the towel and pronounce the victim dead—the decision is left entirely up to the physician running the code. Factors contributing to the decision to stop CPR include the type of heart rhythm, whether the arrest was witnessed, even how old the victim is, but there are no clear algorithms.[3] Some physicians let CPR continue until every medical student has practiced giving compressions. Others go well beyond the 20-minute suggested time limit if the victim is young or otherwise healthy. Still others will cut CPR short if the victim is old and frail, believing they have no real chance at a meaningful recovery.

But at some point, the futility of CPR becomes clear and the doctor running the code calls a time of death. The IVs and intubation tubing are removed, and the victim—the corpse—is dressed in their gown once more. No one pulls a sheet up over their face, but they do close the curtains while the doctor goes to tell the family.

Most deaths in the US are cardiopulmonary deaths. The second type of death, brain death, is both much rarer and more precisely defined.

BRAIN DEATH

When Iva was a teenager, her mother was in a horrible boating accident. Her heart had stopped for over an hour, but because of the cold water, she was treated with Therapeutic Hypothermia. At the time, Iva thought that this meant she was frozen in cryo, like on Star Trek. So, when the doctors rewarmed her, Iva thought she would open her eyes and be fine. Instead, the doctors found no evidence of brain activity, and Iva's mother was pronounced dead.

> Brain death can't be pronounced until the body temperature is AT LEAST 90oF.

Brain Death = Death.

Let me say it again. Brain death is death. It implies the complete absence of brain function. If your character is pronounced brain dead, they are dead, and there is no coming back from it.

Brain death is very clearly defined. Though technically it can be pronounced by any doctor, most of the time brain death is pronounced by a neurologist or neurosurgeon, as they have the most experience with the neurologic exam and testing needed to make the diagnosis.

To diagnose brain death:

- The cause must be known.

- The victim must have stable vital signs, and must not be under the influence of toxins, poisons, or sedating medications

- The victim must be in a coma, with a complete lack of any brainstem reflexes.

> Brainstem reflexes indicate that the lowest, most basic part of the brain is functioning. Without them, the body cannot survive.

- The victim must not initiate breathing on their own.

The diagnosis of brain death requires a thorough physical exam. Just the apnea test–which determines if the victim can initiate breathing on their own– takes 8-10 minutes. If your character is going to be diagnosed as brain dead, expect the physician doing so to be in there and poking around for a while.

Fun fact: brain dead corpses can move (so can those who died of cardiopulmonary reasons, though no one ever seems quite as freaked out by that). If someone taps the knee of your dead patient, their leg will kick forward just like yours would. These reflexes are called spinal reflexes–the signal is relayed through the spinal cord, not the brain–so don't worry, the victim is still dead. But the movements aren't limited to a leg kick; complex spinal reflexes can occur as well. In the "Lazarus Sign", the head of the corpse is turned, causing the arms to bend, folding over the chest like a vampire.[4] If the neck is flexed, all four limbs may jerk off the bed.

> Not all corpses will exhibit complex spinal reflexes. But when they're present, you can bet that someone will use them to try and scare the sh*t out of the med student.

The physical exam and the apnea test are sufficient to diagnose brain death. But if there are any questions, other tests can further support the diagnosis. These include:

- **Brain blood flow:** Without blood flow, the brain is dead. Doctors can use several different imaging techniques (ultrasound, CT angiography, etc.) to prove that no blood is flowing to the brain.
- **EEG:** Measures electrical activity in the brain. To prove brain death, there should be no activity.

> In most states, the surgeon who will perform the organ transplant cannot be the one who pronounces death due to conflict of interest.

Iva hadn't understood how her mother could be dead; all that changed was that a doctor walked into the room, performed an exam, and then she was suddenly dead? She didn't look any different than she had when she was alive. The doctors had given them time to say their goodbyes, then a new doctor, one Iva hadn't seen before, asked Iva's father if her mother would have wanted to be an organ donor. He'd agreed, and her mother was wheeled away to surgery later that day. The next time Iva saw her was at the open casket.

> To donate organs, your character must have been previously healthy, <70 years old, and not engaged in activities such as drug abuse.

When brain death is pronounced, the corpse is not immediately taken off life support. Instead, someone from the transplant team—usually the surgeon or PA—is sent to talk to the family about whether or not the deceased would want to donate their organs. If so, they are kept on life support—a ventilator plus medications to keep their blood pressure and heart rate stable—until the transplant team is ready for the surgery. If the family chooses not to donate, the cadaver will be taken off life support.

> The quick removal from life support is particularly true during the COVID pandemic, when ventilators were in very short supply.

I'm going to say it one more time for good measure: brain dead is dead. If your character is brain dead and is not going to donate organs, they are taken off life support. Period. The family isn't choosing to take your character off life support, and they don't get to ask to keep the corpse on life support until the children or the wife or the parents arrive at the hospital. The person is dead and someone else needs those resources more.

> This is particularly true during the COVID pandemic, when ventilators were in very short supply.

PRONOUNCING DEATH

Finally, Iva has no more tears. She gets to her feet and finds the nurse, informing her that her father has passed. A few minutes later, the hospice doctor arrives. He gives Iva his condolences, listens to her father's heart and lungs with his stethoscope, then pronounces him dead.

Technically, your character isn't dead until they've been pronounced or declared dead. Only doctors (and in some states, nurses) can pronounce death. First responders—police, EMTs, paramedics, firefighters, etc.—declare it. This usually happens when it is *very* clear that the victim is no longer alive. If there's any chance of survival, no matter how slim, first responders will not declare death. Eventually, a doctor will have to sign a death certificate, but first-responders being able to declare someone dead on arrival prevents them from having to do CPR on a rotting corpse.

To pronounce death, a doctor needs to examine your character. They'll confirm their identity, then call their name and perform a sternal rub to confirm that they are unresponsive. Then they'll peel open their eyelids and shine a light into them—the pupils will be dilated and will not constrict with light. They'll check for a pulse at the wrist or neck, then take out their stethoscope to listen for heart and lung sounds. Finally, they will note aloud the victim's name, date, and time of death.[2]

No one teaches doctors how to do this. Doctors, especially residents and interns, can be called to pronounce death in the middle of the night on people they've never met. Pronouncing death is considered a basic task, yet it can be incredibly stressful, especially when the doctor must break the news to the family. It is not at all unusual for the doctor to seem callous, cold, or overly familiar while performing this task.

POST-MORTEM EXAM (AUTOPSY)

The palliative care doctor asks Iva if she would like to request an autopsy, but Iva refuses. She knows it was cancer that killed her father.

The post-mortem exam (also called an autopsy or necropsy) is the examination of the body after death. It is done for one of four reasons:

1. The death was considered suspicious or unexpected.
2. The cause of death was unknown.
3. The cause of death was possibly due to a public health concern.
4. Requested by family.

> In 2020, autopsy numbers spiked due to COVID.[5]

Unlike what you've probably seen on TV, autopsies are quite rare. Autopsy rates have dropped precipitously in the last fifty years; before 1960, about 50% of all deaths ended in an autopsy. This number dropped to below 5% in the 2010s. This decline was caused by a combination of decreased funding–autopsies are generally not covered by insurance–and a loosening of regulations on when autopsies need to be performed.

Autopsies are performed in morgues, usually connected to a hospital. In an autopsy, the pathologist begins with a detailed external inspection. She then makes the famous Y-shaped incision and peels away the skin and fat. Then, she uses a bone saw (or hedge clippers) to cut through the breastbone and ribs. She removes and evaluates the organs, taking tissue samples for later inspection, then places the remainder in a sealed plastic bag. If the brain is examined (it doesn't always have to be), she'll make an incision in the back of the skull, lifting off the skull cap (the round top of the skull) and gently dissect out the brain.[9]

> The cadaver will not smell like formaldehyde, because it has not been preserved. Instead, the cadaver will smell of old blood. When bones are cut, they smell like Fritos.

A cadaver that has undergone autopsy can still have an open casket. The skull cap is replaced and covered by hair. The internal cavity is lined with plastic and the organs—still in their bags—are placed inside. Then the body is sewn back up using the famous baseball stitch and sent to the mortician for dressing and makeup.[9]

STAGES OF DEATH

When Iva returns to her father's room, he looks exactly as he did when he was alive—only a bit paler. His skin is still warm as she brushes aside his thin white hair to plant a last kiss on his wrinkled forehead.

When your character first dies, they won't *look* dead. Stories abound of medical students performing full exams on a corpse they thought was sleeping. At first, corpses look exactly as they did before they died. But they don't stay that way. The four stages of death below do not necessarily occur in order—many occur simultaneously—but together, they can be used to predict the time of death.

PALLOR MORTIS (PALENESS OF DEATH)

Pallor mortis occurs 15-30 minutes after death and is just the corpse turning super pale due to the lack of blood circulation. It's most obvious on pale-skinned people—those with darker skin still get it, but it may be less noticeable, or may come across as more of a gray tint. At this point, the muscles will relax, becoming completely flaccid.

> **Death sh*ts**
>
> Not an official stage of death, but an all-too-frequent occurrence. Death leads to muscle relaxion, including the relaxation of the anal sphincter. All the cr*p that your character hasn't been able to eliminate comes out in one gigantic, stinky rush.

ALGOR MORTIS (COLDNESS OF DEATH)

Algor mortis happens when the body, no longer able to create heat, drops to the temperature of the external environment. It usually takes 18-20 hours for the body to equilibrate to the ambient temperature. Since human flesh loses heat at a predictable rate, pathologists use the temperature of the corpse to calculate the time of death using equations that account for variables such as the ambient air temperature, and the victim's clothing, body mass, and posture.[6] Around this time, the eyes start to look filmy.

RIGOR MORTIS (STIFFNESS OF DEATH)

You've heard of rigor mortis—the stiffening of the muscles of a corpse after death. It occurs because the body has run out of the cell's energy source, ATP. Without ATP, the muscle cells are unable to disengage, locking them in place. It begins 2-4 hours after death, peaks around 12 hours, and continues for 24-48 hours. Because of this wide variability, rigor mortis alone is not a great way to predict the time of death. But it's still very useful to investigators, as the victim will be locked in the position in which they died (or were positioned shortly after death). They'll even retain facial expressions.

LIVOR MORTIS (BLUISH-PURPLE OF DEATH)

Blood is a fluid, so when the heart stops pushing it around, it pools, forming what is essentially a giant bruise in the lowest part of the body. Most of the time—at least in hospitals—people die while lying supine, so the fluid pools in their back and the backs of their arms and thighs. But if your character were to die face down, the blood would pool in their stomach and face.

Livor mortis starts as a bright redness of the skin at around thirty minutes after death. After about six hours, it begins to look more like a bruise. Early on in livor mortis, your character could touch the reddened area of livor mortis and it would blanch white, meaning that the blood hadn't clotted yet. But after twelve hours or so, the blood becomes "fixed," meaning that it won't blanch, and if the victim were to be repositioned, the blood wouldn't move.

Supine = face up
Prone = face down

VERY, VERY, VERY APPROXIMATE STAGES OF DEATH BY TIME

Temperature	Tone	Blood Pooling	Time from Death
Warm	Flaccid	No	<3 hours
Warm	Stiff	Blanchable	3-8 hours
Cool	Stiff	Blanchable	8-12 hours
Cool	Stiff	Non-blanchable	12-18 hours
Cold	Stiff	Non-blanchable	18-36 hours
Cold	Not stiff	Non-blanchable	>36 hours

CLICHÉ: LAST WORDS

"I am dying"

Cough cough

"Let me take the next twenty minutes to muse aloud about the meaning of life, love, and our beautiful relationship."

There is a veritable trove of tropes surrounding last words. But in all of them, the victim is totally conscious and cogent. They might be breathing hard, covered in gore, and coughing up blood, but they're with it enough to look their loved one (or nemesis) in the eye and tell them that it's been an honor, or that they loved them, or to take care of the dog when they're gone. Then they sigh, and look away, their eyes going glassy.

I've never seen a death that looks anything like this. Most in-hospital deaths follow the stages of dying laid out earlier in the chapter. By the time your character is ready to die, they'll likely have been unconscious for hours (days?), their rattling breaths getting further and further apart until there are no more breaths at all. They usually aren't conscious enough to know who they are, never mind compose coherent and meaningful last words.

That doesn't mean you can't give your character a lucid interval in which to have these important conversations. That would be both realistic and appropriate; it just wouldn't happen *right* as they die. At the moment of death, they probably wouldn't be coherent (or conscious) enough to do it then.

The exception, of course, is trauma. Traumatic wounds causing exsanguination take seconds to minutes (depending on the wound) before your character would lose consciousness. And if the knife/bullet to the chest caused a cardiac tamponade or hemothorax, they could certainly have time for a few last words. H*ll, studies have shown that animals retain consciousness for up to thirty seconds after decapitation,[7] so you could go full-on Anne Boleyn for your character's last words if you were so inclined.

PART 4: Q&A

THE TOP 10 QUESTIONS I GET FROM WRITERS

1. **One of my characters is injured while they're out in the woods/desert/somewhere far from help. What are some stopgap measures my MC can use to save their life?**

This could be a whole book in and of itself, so I'm going to keep it brief.

Sprains: Treat with RICE: Rest, Ice, Ibuprofen (or other anti-inflammatory medication), and Elevation. If your character needs to walk on a sprained ankle, an improvised splint (see below) may help.

Broken bones: First, align the limb by pulling slowly and gently until the bone is in proper anatomic alignment. This will hurt like h*ll, but your character will feel much better once the bone is aligned. Second, immobilize the limb. If it's an arm, that means making a sling with whatever extra clothing is lying around. If it's a leg, your character can use hiking poles (or the straightest, sturdiest sticks they can find) to fashion a splint, padding them generously before tying them in place around the injured area. After splinting, make sure your character still has a pulse at their wrist or foot. If not, or if the limb is going numb, the splint is too tight.

> Splints should be BUFF: Big, Ugly, Fat, and Fluffy.

Move the limb as little as possible–this will probably mean fashioning a litter to drag them. Make sure your character is looking out for signs of shock, particularly if they broke their femur. And if bone is poking out through skin, keep the area clean and touch it as infrequently as possible.

> Splints that are too tight cut off blood flow and can cause tissue death.

Lacerations (cuts): The first step is to control bleeding by applying pressure. Sterile gauze is best, but extra clothing can work in a pinch. Superglue can also work for smaller cuts. Once the bleeding stops, flush the wound with CLEAN water (from a moving stream, not from a standing pool) and apply a bandage–again, sterile gauze is best, but anything that can both occlude the wound and provide some pressure (i.e., a shirt tied tight around the area) is good enough.

But what if the laceration is super deep, or the bleeding just won't stop? Your character can try suturing it closed, though they'll need a needle and thread. Making sure both needle and thread are sterilized is vitally important, particularly if your character isn't heading to the hospital anytime soon. Needles can be sterilized by boiling them for 30 minutes or holding them over a flame until the metal glows red. Thread is both harder and more important to sterilize since it's the part that stays in the body. If your character doesn't have a suture kit–complete with sterilized thread–on them, I'd have your character hold off on suturing anything.

Tourniquets are only used in cases of life-threatening hemorrhage, but if someone is bleeding out from an extremity, your character shouldn't hesitate to use one. If your character needs to tie a tourniquet, they need to tie something very tight above the level of the wound; tight enough that they can no longer feel a pulse in that extremity. This is hard to do, particularly if your character doesn't happen to carry a commercial tourniquet around with them. Improvised tourniquets are not as effective–but if they're all your character has, it'll have to be enough. Tourniquets require three parts: a band, a winch, and a securing mechanism. The band wraps around the extremity and should be wide–belts and zip ties are too narrow. Ties, bandanas, or even a pant leg will work. Once the band is in place, it's wrapped around the winch and pulled tight. A sturdy stick (at least the diameter of a broom) works as a makeshift winch; your character will use it to pull the band tighter and tighter. Once it's as tight as physically possible, the band must be secured in place using a hair tie, rubber band, or even a key ring.[1]

Bullet wounds: Pack the wound to stop the bleeding. Sterilized gauze is best if they have it, but anything to stuff into the wound to stop the bleeding is better than nothing. For small entrance wounds, tampons can work in a pinch. They're sterile, and many women carry one on them.

> Don't worry about digging out the bullet.

2. How can I make my character pass out from blood loss without killing them?

I often see writers writing scenes of their character being cut/shot/otherwise beat up, losing consciousness due to blood loss, then waking up some time later, alone. This drives me crazy. Your character isn't going to stop bleeding just because they passed out. If they are bleeding fast enough to pass out, they are bleeding fast enough to die. It doesn't take much to go from unconscious to dead.

Remember the 10-20-30% rule?[2]

- 10% blood loss: No symptoms

- 20% blood loss: Dizziness and Anxiety
- 30% blood loss: Shock
- 40% blood loss: Unconsciousness
- 50% blood loss: Death

Your character loses about 40% of their blood before they lose consciousness, but only another 10%–just ¼ of what they've already lost–to die. This means that you have a very narrow window between your character passing out and them dying. In between, something has to stop the bleeding. And that means medical care.

If your character is slowly leaking from a dozen different wounds, it might be enough to have someone throw on a bunch of bandages and apply pressure. But most of the time, if your character is bleeding out, it means an artery was severed or an internal organ crushed.

Bleeding from the large arteries in the groin, wrist, and neck are hard to stop. Your character can use a tourniquet to slow it down (see above), but the definitive treatment is going to be surgery. Internal bleeding, either arterial or from a lacerated solid organ such as the liver, is even more difficult to stop without surgery. If your character needs to save someone who is bleeding out, they'll have to act quickly to stop the bleeding before the victim loses too much blood.

> Don't use a tourniquet on the neck. That's called strangulation.

The first step is to staunch the bleeding as best they can, using a tourniquet or bandages plus pressure. Next, they need to get the victim's blood pressure up by giving fluids, blood products, and medications to constrict the blood vessels. But these are only temporary solutions; the definitive treatment is to go in there and physically tie off or cauterize the blood vessels–in other words, surgery.

If your character passes out from blood loss and someone doesn't immediately perform the above steps, your character is dead. So, if you want them to be left in a cave for dead, find another reason for them to lose consciousness.

3. What injuries would be realistic after getting beaten up?

Pretty much anything. I know that isn't a very satisfying answer but hear me out. The extent of your characters' injuries depends on so many factors that I, without intimate knowledge of your story, can't reasonably tell you the exact extent of your characters' injuries.

Let's say your character gets stabbed in the abdomen. Depending on the length/sharpness of the weapon, the exact location of the wound, the angle of entry/exit, the force exerted, even how much fat your character carries around their middle, the injury could range from a mere flesh wound to nearly instantly fatal. Yes, some injuries are more likely than others, but you, the author, have a lot of leeway here. It's your story. As long as you stay within the realm of reasonable, you can do what you want.

A few caveats:

- If your character is hit on the head hard enough for them to be unconscious for more than a few seconds, they're going to have some brain damage. Even if they're unconscious for just a few seconds, they're going to have a concussion. If they're out for more than 20 minutes, they probably have major, permanent brain damage.

- If your character passes out from blood loss, they're going to die of blood loss if they aren't treated soon (see Question #3).

- You can't put weight on a broken bone. I don't care how manly your character is, he's not going anywhere if he broke his leg.

- Yes, gut wounds cause infection, but not for a few days. The more immediate concern is still blood loss.

> The exception is small, hairline fractures or stress fractures of the ankle and the fibula.

- Your character will only cough up blood if their lungs, trachea, mouth, nose, or esophagus are bleeding. Stop having your character cough up blood after being punched in the gut.

- Stop wrenching broken noses back into place; your character is liable to do more damage than good. Nasal bones are bones and, like any other bone, they should be set by someone who knows what they're doing. Bad breaks may even require surgery. Unless the break is making it difficult for your character to breathe, have them ice it and take Tylenol until they're able to get to a medical professional (or a boxing coach) to sort it out.

- Canes are used on the opposite side of the body. If your character's left leg is injured, they'll use a cane on the right.

4. What are the recovery times for…?

How long will it take my character to recover from being stabbed in the gut? From a broken arm? From a heart attack?

These are all great questions, but they are very difficult to answer. Recovery times vary widely based on the type and severity of injury or illness as well as your character's demographics and overall health. This means that similar injuries can have remarkably different recovery times as well as overall outcomes.

Let's say your character breaks their femur–the long bone of their leg. Femurs are sturdy bones, so it takes a lot of force to break one. If your character is young and otherwise healthy, they might recover in as little as 3 months. But if your frail, elderly character gets the same fracture, it might take as much as 12 months for them to heal. Or they'll never recover at all; they'll be admitted to the hospital for surgical repair but then develop one complication after another–blood clots, pneumonia, infection–until they finally succumb and pass away. It's more common than you'd think; studies have shown that the elderly are more than twice as likely to die in the year following a hip fracture.[1]

> If your character is injured, they shouldn't drive until they are no longer taking prescription-strength painkillers (like opioids).

Never fear–I'm still going to make a list of approximate recovery times for a bunch of different ailments. I just want to be very clear that these are *approximate* recovery times. Characters who are old, frail, or have concurrent medical conditions (like diabetes) are more likely to be on the long end of these ranges, while children and healthy young characters are likely to be on the shorter end.

INJURIES

- **Sprained ankle:** 2 weeks (mild sprain) to 6 months (severe sprain).
- **Broken leg (tibia-fibula fracture):** 6 weeks in a cast, 3-6 months to recovery.
- **Broken leg (femur fracture):** 2-3 months in a cast/traction, 3-12 months to recovery.
- **Broken finger:** 4-6 weeks.
- **Broken arm/wrist (radius-ulna fracture):** 6-8 weeks.
- **Dislocated shoulder:** 2-3 days in a sling. 2-6 months to recovery.

SUTURE REMOVAL:

- **Face & scalp:** 5-7 days
- **Trunk & arms:** 10-14 days
- **Legs:** 2-3 weeks

> Many sutures, colloquially called stitches, are made of dissolvable thread, and do not need to be taken out.

TRAUMA

- **Burns (severe):** Estimate 1 day in the hospital for every 1% of your character's body that is burned.

- **Gunshot wounds**: HIGHLY variable, based on the location of the wound, gun type, etc.
    - May take a year or more to return to normal functioning.

- **Penetrating abdominal trauma (stabbings, gunshot wounds, etc.):** 3-6 days in the hospital plus 4-6 months recovery.
    - One study found that one-third of all patients with penetrating abdominal trauma died of their wounds.[2]

- **Concussion:** 7-14 days; a post-concussive syndrome may last much longer.

- **Traumatic Brain Injury**: Fastest improvement happens in the first 6 months. Many never return to baseline functioning.
    - One study found that two years after brain injury, 30% still needed assistance with daily living, 25% had depression, and 70% could not hold a job.[3]

SURGERIES

- **Appendectomy (routine):** 1-2 days in the hospital; 2-4 weeks recovery at home.
    - If appendix burst, 5-7 days in the hospital.

- **Coronary Artery Bypass Graft (CABG):** 5-7 days in the hospital. Walk after 3 days. Cardiac rehabilitation for approximately 12 weeks.

- **Coronary Stent (Cardiac Catheterization):** 12-24 hours in the hospital, outpatient cardiac rehabilitation for 4-8 weeks.

- **Cholecystectomy (Gallbladder removal):** 2 weeks recovery at home.

> After cardiac surgeries, your character will be instructed to refrain from sports, driving, straining on the toilet, and sex, for at least a week.

- **Organ transplant:** Average hospital stay ranges from 7 days for kidney transplants to 52 days for intestinal transplants.[4]

ILLNESSES

- **Depression:** At least 6 weeks before medications can start to improve mood. Electroconvulsive therapy (ECT) begins to work after just 6-12 treatments (2-6 weeks).[3]

- **Myocardial Infarction (Heart attack):** 1-3 months to return to normal activities.

- **Pneumonia**: 1 week-1 month to return to feeling normal.

5. **Could my character still have sex after being wounded?**

It's not just romance writers; authors of all genres seem to have a thing for having their characters get down and dirty right after a fight scene. And that's perfectly plausible; studies have shown a definite link between high adrenaline states and increased arousal.[1] But if your character is seriously wounded, sexy time could be downright painful. Below, I've compiled a list of injuries and illnesses that might impede your character's ability to do the nasty.

> These estimates are for penis-in-vagina intercourse. Other types of sex, particularly oral sex and mutual masturbation are much less likely to cause pain or discomfort.

- **Abdominal Trauma or Surgery:** Major trauma to the abdomen, including gunshot wounds and anything requiring abdominal surgery, can be a contraindication for sex. And while there isn't a lot of data available for the timing of sex after abdominal trauma/surgery, the general recommendation is to wait a week or two, then proceed gently.

- **Childbirth (vaginal or C-section):** 4-6 weeks.

- **Gender Affirming Surgery:** 12 weeks for vulvoplasty (male-to-female reassignment surgery). 6 weeks after stage 3 phalloplasty (female-to-male reassignment).

- **Heart attack or Cardiac Arrest:** Depends on the severity of the attack, ranging from a few weeks to several months.
    o If your character can walk up two flights of stairs without difficulty, they can have sex.

- **Hip fracture:** No sexual activity for 4-6 weeks.

- **Limb injuries:** Broken, sprained, or lacerated limbs shouldn't be a hindrance to sex, provided your characters can utilize positions that don't put any pressure on the injury.

> Return to sex after miscarriage or abortion can be very difficult. Your character might not be emotionally ready for a much longer time than she is physically able to have intercourse.

- **Miscarriage or abortion:** After the woman has stopped bleeding.
- **Traumatic Brain Injury:** There's no rule as to how long your character needs to wait to have intercourse after being knocked on the head. But about 50% of people with head injuries experience a significant decrease in their sex drive after the event.[4] Many others experience problems achieving an erection or orgasm.

6. **How do I poison my character? I want something tasteless, smell-less, and instantaneously lethal that won't degrade if it's baked/cooked/boiled/eaten.**

Funnily enough, they didn't teach poisoning in medical school. If you're looking for plants to poison your characters with, you'd be better off talking to an avid gardener. However, there are a few famous plants and animals that make some stellar natural poisons.

Digoxin: A cardiac medication that increases the contractile strength of the heart, is made from the Foxglove plant. Normally, it's used in people with heart failure. In high doses, it causes GI upset, heart palpitations, trouble breathing, and fainting. Interestingly, your character may notice yellow-green discoloration in their vision–a sure sign of digoxin toxicity. However, it's pretty hard to die from overdose on the medication, never mind from ingesting the flower itself.

Tetrodotoxin (TTX): A toxin derived from pufferfish, TTX prevents nerves from firing and causes increasing paralysis throughout the body. If your character ingests TTX, they will feel numbness and tingling in their lips and mouth that spreads across their body. Once the toxin reaches the diaphragm–the muscle required to breathe–they will asphyxiate. Without treatment, your character will die, fully conscious but unable to draw breath. It isn't a pretty way to go.

The toxin is heat stable, meaning it doesn't break down when cooked, and incredibly lethal–more than 1,000x more toxic than cyanide.[5] Fugu–a Japanese delicacy–is raw pufferfish specially prepared to remove the sources of TTX. It takes years of training to learn to prepare fugu, but people still die from TTX poisoning every year.[5] It's also important to note that pufferfish are not the only animals that produce this toxin; TTX can be produced by certain species of octopi, flatworm, even the rough-skinned newts native to the Pacific Northwest.

There is no known antidote to TTX.

Honey: You've probably heard the story about oleander honey; an old woman sells honey made from the flowers of oleander plants and the victims die from the poisoned honey. However, as far as I can tell, this is just a myth. Oleander flowers do not produce nectar, so bees don't make honey from them. However, oleander can be deadly if you eat the leaves or flowers, though you'd have to eat quite a bit.

But if you want to poison someone with honey, you don't have to go to all the trouble of trying to feed the bees a particular type of flower. Instead, just give the victim raw honey–your character can buy it in the "health food" aisle at the grocery store! Raw honey can contain the spores of the bacteria that produce botulinum toxin, a paralytic toxin that prevents nerves from firing. Without treatment, your character will asphyxiate. There is a catch though; botulism from honey is usually contracted by children less than one year old. The bigger and older your character is, the less likely they are to get botulism from honey. If you want to give an adult botulism, either have them eat some improperly canned food or inoculate a wound. The most common source of wound botulism is contaminated drugs, particularly tar heroin, though your character could also get it from a nasty traumatic wound like road rash.

> Honey poisoning, also known as Mad Honey, is real, though rare. Caused by grayanotoxins in honey made from rhododendron flowers, it causes changes to the heart rhythm, respiratory depression, nausea/vomiting and dizziness.[6] It is rarely fatal.

7. **What are some chronic diseases/conditions that can make my character appear 'weak'?**

First, people with chronic conditions aren't weak; they've often had to overcome incredible obstacles and have come out stronger for it. Second, if you don't have at least a general idea of what disease your character has, you probably shouldn't give them one. Let me explain:

Question 1: "I need my character to be a wheelchair user. They weren't born needing a wheelchair, but they didn't have an accident either–I need it to be an illness that came on when they were in their 20's or 30's. What are some conditions that can cause this?"

Question 2: "What conditions could put my character in a wheelchair?"

The first example is specific; it shows a character who was once able to walk but is now a wheelchair user. It indicates that this character's condition–whatever it may be–is an integral part of the story. The second example shows that all that really matters is the wheelchair; the writer hasn't put much thought into the character sitting in it. Don't be this person.

Giving your protagonist a chronic condition can certainly add depth to their character, but I caution you against doing so lightly. It will require a lot of research that is outside the scope of this book. People with chronic conditions tend to know a lot about their illness, which means you're going to need a solid grasp of the medical details. And to avoid stereotyping your character, you'll also need to gain a deeper understanding of the culture of chronic illness and disability. Ever heard of the Spoon Theory? Inspiration porn? "Supercrips"? If you're going to give a character a chronic condition or disability, you're going to need to get familiar with these terms and others.

Avoid clichés like the plague (see what I did there?). But seriously. There are so many clichés and tropes surrounding disability and chronic illness–albino villains, crippled geniuses, evil eunuchs, emotionless autistics, fakers of chronic pain, swearing Tourette's–the list goes on. Make sure you aren't accidentally falling into them.

And finally: people with chronic illnesses and disabilities are people first. Your character shouldn't get all moony-eyed because someone treated them like a human or be treated as an inspiration just for existing. And if you're creating a character whose sole purpose in the story is the be the 'sick one'–please, just stop.

8. What does it mean to be catatonic?

If I had a penny for every time I've heard someone misuse the word catatonic, I'd have… about $2. But that's a lot of pennies! People seem to think that catatonic is synonymous with being unresponsive, or that the only way for someone in catatonia to behave is for them to lie flat in bed staring up at the ceiling. Neither is true.

Catatonia is a complex medical condition associated with several different mental illnesses, including schizophrenia, depression, and bipolar disorder. Medical conditions, like stroke or Parkinson's Disease, can also cause catatonia. It is characterized by a combination of psychiatric, language, and motor features.[7]

- **Altered Level of Consciousness**
    - **Stupor:** Your character does not move or react to their environment, even though their eyes are open, and they are conscious. The presence of stupor indicates a severe form of catatonia.
    - **Agitation:** For no apparent reason, your character becomes agitated or excited.

- **Automatic Obedience:** Your character automatically obeys every instruction.
- **Imitation**
    - **Echolalia:** Imitating another person's speech; echoing a word.

- o **Echopraxia:** Imitating another's movements.
- **Language Changes**
    - o **Mutism:** Your character doesn't speak or has trouble talking.
    - o **Verbigeration:** Obsessive repetition of non-meaningful words.
    - o **Word Salad:** Rapid-fire, incoherent speech (gibberish).
- **Movement Changes**
    - o **Grimacing:** Unusual facial movements for no apparent reason.
    - o **Stereotypy:** Repetitive, purposeless movements.
    - o **Mannerisms:** Repetitive movements that initially had meaning, such as repeated saluting or grasping as if to shake a hand.
- **Postural Changes**
    - o **Waxy Flexibility:** Slight resistance to movement by the examiner.
    - o **Posturing:** Your character will strike a pose and stay there, perhaps for hours. An extreme version is **Catalepsy,** in which the limbs are rigid and remain in position even against force.
    - o **Negativism:** Your character will resist any attempts to move their body, reacting with the same amount of force given (i.e., if the examiner pushes harder, they push back with the same strength).

Your character doesn't have to exhibit all of these symptoms; several, such as mutism and echolalia, are contradictory. If you want your character to be catatonic, you only need three of these symptoms.[7] The most common signs of catatonia are stupor and mutism.

9. **How much damage could a corrupt doctor do?**

Historically, there have been some straight-up evil doctors. Nazi doctors like Josef Mengele and Claud Clauberg, are the first that come to mind, but Nazis don't have a monopoly on sadism. Dr. James Marion Sims–considered the "father of modern gynecology"–conducted his research on enslaved black women, without their consent or anesthesia. Dr. Walter Freeman, who had no surgical training, pioneered the lobotomy using a literal ice pick. There have been multiple serial killers, mob doctors, back-alley abortionists, and doctors who killed patients to acquire their property.[8]

While it's easy to focus on these terrifying examples, it's more difficult to rise to these levels of evil in modern American medicine. Most of these doctors practiced in the days before licensing boards or oversight committees, when home visits were the norm. Several of the most horrific examples practiced during periods where whole groups of people were considered subhuman and were not given even the basics of human rights. Theoretically, the practice of medicine has learned from these egregious mistakes and taken steps to prevent such evil from rearing its ugly head again.

First, medicine has seriously curbed the power of the individual doctor. With the rise of advanced practitioners and multidisciplinary healthcare teams, doctors have become accustomed to working in teams, receiving feedback, and responding appropriately. In the OR, for example, any member of the surgical team–from the attending surgeon to the scrub tech–is legally obligated to call a "time out" if they think anything inappropriate or incorrect is about to happen. This isn't to say that a doctor can't act inappropriately–I once had a surgeon throw a bloody scalpel at me– but that it's harder for doctors to get away with bad behavior when the people around them are empowered to speak up. That doctor who threw the scalpel at me was reported by one of the nurses, and he was banned from working with students for several years.

Second, doctors must document absolutely everything they do. With the ubiquity of electronic medical records (EMRs), this means that every drug they've ever prescribed, every procedure they've performed, and every patient they've consulted with is recorded. Any mysterious deaths will leave a paper trail so large it could be seen from space. The statistics from these EMRs are closely watched by both their employer and state/federal agencies. If a doctor's prescribing patterns don't match up to her peers, then it will set off a red flag.

Theoretically.

Of course, we know this system doesn't always work. The opioid epidemic is proof that doctors can get away with overprescribing potentially deadly and addictive medications. Some doctors went so far as setting up "pill mills"–prescribing opioids to anyone who could pay cash for the prescription. And while many of these physicians were caught and their licenses revoked, it's difficult to imagine that no one is continuing this practice under the table.

The other way the system can fail to stop corrupt doctors is if the system itself is corrupt. Doctors have participated in some horrible civil programs. In the 1970s, physicians sterilized Native American Women without their understanding or consent.[9] In 2020, women in the ICE detention facilities were sterilized in a similar fashion.[10] These doctors were acting legally, but the morality of their actions leaves much to be desired.

10. **How does the US healthcare system work?**

While writers may not ask this question in so many words, their lack of understanding shows through in their writing. And it's understandable to be confused; the healthcare system in the United States is super messed up. Pretty much everyone agrees that our healthcare system is more expensive and less effective than pretty much any other developed country in the world.[11] I'm not here to get political, but the sh*tty healthcare system in the US is a veritable trove of sources of external conflict if you know where to look.

> It's impossible for me to answer this question without straying into my personal opinions. If you want to avoid anything political, just skip this question and move on.

EMPLOYER-BASED HEALTH INSURANCE

You probably know that the US healthcare system is based on a network of private insurance companies. Your character buys insurance through a company that contracts out to specific clinics and hospital groups. When your character needs care, they go to those in-network providers, who in turn bill the insurance companies.

Most people get their health insurance through their employer. They still pay for their health insurance, but at a much lower rate than if they tried to get insurance on their own. But what about people who are unemployed, self-employed, retired, in school, or working for an employer who doesn't offer health insurance? That's where the public programs come in.

> The employee-based health insurance system means that if your character loses their job, they also lose access to medical care–both for themselves and for their family!

GOVERNMENT-SUBSIDIZED HEALTH INSURANCE

Contrary to what you might have heard, government-subsidized healthcare is alive and well in the US. Traditionally, it comes in two main forms: Medicare and Medicaid. **Medicare** is a government health insurance system available for all people over sixty-five, as well as some people with disabilities and terminal illnesses. **Medicaid** is the government health insurance system for low-income individuals, particularly children, pregnant women, and people living off social security.

> Medical expenses are the #1 cause of bankruptcy in the US.[12]

If you want to trap your character in the cycle of poverty, consider giving them a chronic illness (not a disability) and a low-wage job; they won't be able to get a raise or higher paying job without losing their Medicaid eligibility, but the increased earnings wouldn't be enough to pay for healthcare. It's a catch-22 faced by many Americans. If you want to tug at the heartstrings, give the chronic illness to their child.

GOVERNMENT MARKETPLACE

What about the people who don't have insurance through their employer but also don't qualify for Medicaid or Medicare? Well, up until 2010, they were pretty much SOL. Buying private, unsubsidized insurance is horrifically expensive, with high monthly premiums and even higher deductibles. People with chronic illnesses—those who needed healthcare the most—were targeted for higher premiums, and pre-existing medical conditions were generally not covered at all.

Since affordable, comprehensive health insurance was out of reach for many people, they avoided going to the doctor unless it was an emergency, getting care through the Emergency Department only when the situation became so dire that they had no other choice. This lack of access to health insurance drove up the cost of healthcare, increased ED wait times, widened racial and economic inequities, and even caused a significant number of deaths. You might think I'm being dramatic, but a 2008 study found that over 26,000 Americans died each year because they didn't have health insurance.[14]

In 2010, the Affordable Care Act also known as the ACA or "Obamacare," sought to increase access to healthcare by creating government-subsidized health insurance plans for people who were unable to purchase it through their employer. The system is stupidly complicated, but the basic idea is that each state sets up a "Marketplace" where your character can go to buy health insurance that is subsidized at rates similar to that of private employers. The ACA had mixed success, to put it nicely, but the rates of uninsured and underinsured individuals have decreased significantly in the last decade.[15]

THE BOTTOM LINE

If your character interacts with the healthcare system—whether they have a car accident or a chronic illness—their access to insurance very much needs to be at the front of their mind. Without some sort of insurance, they won't be able to access the healthcare they need. And while Emergency Departments can't turn anyone away due to EMTALA, clinics, surgeons, and imaging centers certainly can. In real life, dealing with insurance is messy and frustrating; in your writing, it can be a source of external tension that pulls your character down a dark path.

APPENDIX 1: PARTS OF A HOSPITAL

THE PARTS OF THE HOSPITAL range from intensive care wards to conference rooms. Not every hospital will have every type of floor; bigger, teaching hospitals are more likely to have more specialized floors and space dedicated to research laboratories and large conference rooms. Smaller, rural hospitals are more likely to be limited to general medicine and surgical floors.

- Administration: Offices, conference rooms, classrooms, etc.
- Catheterization Laboratory (Cath Lab)
- Dialysis Unit
- Emergency Department (ED)

FLOORS:

- Cardiac Care Unit/Cardiothoracic Unit (CCU/CTU)
- General Medicine
- General Surgery
- Geriatric
- Isolation Ward
- Labor & Delivery (L&D)
- Mother-baby Unit
    o Sometimes called Postpartum Suites
- Neurology
- Neurosurgery
- Oncology: Cancer Wards
    o Gyn-Onc: For gynecologic cancers
    o Ped-Onc: Pediatric cancer
    o Rad-Onc: For patients recovering from radiation therapy.

> L&D consists of birthing suites and an OR for emergency C-sections.

> L&D and Postpartum floors often have the nicest rooms in the hospital.

A WRITER'S GUIDE TO MEDICINE

- Orthopedic Surgery
- Pediatric
- Plastic surgery
- Renal (kidney disease)
- Hospice/Palliative Care
- ICU: Intensive Care Units
    - Burn Unit
    - Cardiac ICU (CICU)
    - Medical ICU (MICU)
    - Neonatal ICU (NICU)
    - Neurology ICU
    - Pediatric ICU (PICU)
    - Surgical ICU (SICU)
    - Trauma ICU (TICU)
- Lab
- Morgue
- Medical Imaging
- Observation Unit (Obs)
- Operating Room or Operating Theater (OR)
- Pharmacy
- Post-Anesthesia Care Unit (PACU)
- Pre-Operation Area (Pre-Op)
- Psychiatric ward
- Rehabilitation Area
- Step-Down Units (SDUs)

> All wards have the capability to handle individual patients that need some level of isolation, but sometimes entire wards need to be set aside for isolation (i.e., COVID wards)

> Psychiatric wards are locked units, separated from the rest of the hospital.

APPENDIX 2: MEDICAL EQUIPMENT 101

BASIC EQUIPMENT

- Bed pads ("Chucks")
    - Disposable liners for hospital beds and exam tables

- Biohazard containment
    - Marked red bags for disposal of human tissue or fluids.

- Blood pressure cuff (sphygmomanometer)
    - Cuff that tightens around upper arm to measure blood pressure
    - Can be automatic or manual

- Hospital Gown
    - May be cloth (long-term wear) or paper (single use)

- Pulse Oximeter
    - Small device that clips to finger, toe, or earlobe and uses light to measure your character's pulse and oxygenation of their blood.

- Sharps containers
    - Red plastic bin for disposing of needles.
    - Will be one in every room

- Stethoscope
    - Two-sided bell with a single tube connecting to plastic-tipped earpieces
    - Used to listen to heart, lungs, blood vessels, and abdomen.

INPATIENT EQUIPMENT

- Commode
    - Mobile toilet used for patients who cannot easily get to the bathroom
    - Looks like a chair with a bucket under the seat

- Computer on Wheels OR Workstation on Wheels (COW/WOW)
    - Wheeled, standing computer.
    - Drawers (may be locked) with equipment
        - Wound care, intubation supplies, etc.

- Crash Cart
    - Wheeled cart (usually red) stocked with medications and medical devices needed to provide advanced life support

- Emesis basin
    - Stainless steel or plastic shallow basin for puking. Shaped like a kidney bean.

- Gurney
    - Height-adjustable wheeled bed used for medical transport

- Intermittent Pneumatic Compression Device (IPCs)
    - Inflatable cuffs that go around your character's calves
    - Inflate and deflate periodically.
    - Used to prevent the formation of clots in the leg.

- Infusion pump
    - Controls the flow of fluids from IV bag
    - Small machine attached to IV pole with buttons and number
    - Beeps a lot.

- Patient lifts
    - Large sling suspended by poles over bed (can be manual or electronic).
    - Assists in moving and transferring patients.

- Patient Monitor

- o Screen beside the bed that shows heart rate, breathing rate, blood pressure, and oxygenation.
- o Connected to BP cuff and pulse oximeter.
- o If heart rhythm is present, see Telemetry Monitor
- Suction Canister and Pump
    - o Clear container with fluid level management placed low on character's bed.
    - o May or may not be attached to vacuum pump
    - o Used to suction fluid from lungs, wounds, or surgical sites.

IMAGING

- CT Scan (**C**omputed **T**omography Scan)
    - o Primary instrument used to get clear, detailed images of organs in the abdomen, chest, and blood vessels.
    - o Used after head trauma to look for blood on the brain.
    - o Basically a 3D X-ray
    - o Machine looks like a huge white donut with a narrow table that slides in and out of the hole
    - o Makes a soft whirring noise
    - o Exams take 10-30 minutes.
    - o Higher dose radioactivity.
- MRI (**M**agnetic **R**esonance **I**maging)
    - o Used to generate a detailed 3D image of soft tissue, such as joints, muscle, organs, blood vessels, and brain.
    - o Uses a magnetic field (no exposure to radiation).
    - o Similar to CT, the MRI machine looks like a huge white donut with a narrow table that slides in and out of the hole
    - o LOUD! Bangs, whirs, beeps, knocks, etc., at decibels ranging from a vacuum cleaner to a jet engine.
    - o Exams take anywhere from 15-90 minutes.

- Positron Emission Tomography (PET) Scan
    - Used to detect cancer, heart disease, and brain disease.
    - Radioactive tracer injected
    - Test takes about two hours.

- Ultrasound
    - Used to image the heart, blood vessels, and fetal development.
    - Computer on wheeled table with probes of different sizes and gel.
    - Uses sound waves to look at structures.
    - Doppler: hear whoosh of heartbeat/pulse

- X-ray
    - Looks at differences in density/particularly good for bones (fractures) and lungs
    - Chest X-ray (CXR) looks for pneumonia, lung mass, collapsed lung, etc.
    - "Quick and dirty" –first step in imaging.
    - Low dose radioactivity

CARDIAC

- Echocardiogram
    - Uses sound waves for detailed, dynamic imaging of the heart.
    - Rolling cart with computer, ultrasound probes, and gel.

- ECG Machine (**E**lectro**c**ardio**g**ram)
    - Synonymous with EKG
    - Rolling cart with computer that connects to ECG wires and prints out paper ECG.
    - EKG wires: 10 wires of various colors stuck on your character's chest.

- ECMO (**E**xtra**c**orporeal **M**embrane **O**xygenation)
    - Machine that bypasses heart and lungs to oxygenate patients' blood.
    - Only seen on very ill patients who cannot breathe at all.

- o Wheeled machine with screen connected by red and blue tubing to patient through cannulas in groin and just above collarbone.

- Telemetry Monitor
    - o Patient Monitor that also shows heart rhythm
    - o Connected to three wires (red, black, and white) on character's chest (R chest, L chest, and under L breast).

FIELD MEDICINE

- AED (**A**utomated **E**xternal **D**efibrillator)
    - o Provides instructions for defibrillation ("shocks") during CPR
    - o Found in all public settings–malls, schools, airports, etc.

- Backboard
    - o Rigid board used to lift and move characters with potential spinal injury.

- Bag Valve Mask (BVM)
    - o Inflatable bag used to deliver rescue breaths during CPR.
    - o Sometimes called Ambo bag

- C-collar
    - o Hard plastic collar to stabilize the neck

- Defibrillator
    - o Portable device with sticky pads and wires connecting to chest.
    - o Generates EKG, delivers shock.

- Laryngoscope
    - o Used to intubate.
    - o Silver instrument with long, thin "blade" to hold back the tongue.

- Stretcher
    - o Narrow, wheeled bed with collapsible legs, so it can be loaded into the ambulance.

> Technically, **gurneys** are found in hospitals while **stretchers** are found on ambulances, but the terms are often used interchangeably.

GASTROINTESTINAL

- Colostomy bag
    - Plastic bag that collects thin, watery stool.
    - Usually sits on abdomen.
    - Should not smell bad.
- Nasogastric tube (NG tube)
    - Temporary feeding tube.
    - Long, thin tube placed into the stomach via a nostril.
- PEG Tube/G-Tube
    - More permanent feeding tube.
    - Looks like a small plastic button inserted just below the character's belly button.

HEAD, EYES, EARS, NOSE & THROAT (HEENT)

- Ophthalmoscope
    - Instrument used to look into eyes.
    - Silver handle with bulbous black head with gears on edges and light in the center
- Otoscope
    - Instrument used to look into ears.
    - Silver handle with black head and disposable black plastic tips.

NEUROLOGY

- Electroencephalogram (EEG)
    - Used to look for seizures
    - Evaluates the electrical activity of the brain
    - 25 electrodes glued to the head: long prep time, hair is gross afterward

> EEG requires a lot of prep time. Afterwards, your character's hair will be gross and sticky from the glue.

- Penlight
    - Pocket-sized flashlight used to shine into patient's eyes
    - Used to evaluate pupil size and reactivity
    - Uneven pupils = red flag for impending brain herniation
- Tuning forks
    - Forked silver instrument, like a musical tuning fork
    - Used to look for nerve damage in the hands and feet

ORTHOPEDICS

- Cast
    - Custom-made from plaster to affix broken limb in place.
    - Completely encloses limb and must be removed with a saw.
- Splint
    - Plastic and/or fabric partially encircling limb to provide stabilization
- Traction devices
    - Slings, weights, and pulleys attached to the hospital bed to keep a joint or broken bone in position.

RESPIRATORY

- Endotracheal (ET)/Nasotracheal (NT) tubing
    - Rigid plastic tubing used for intubation.
- Face mask
    - Clear plastic mask used to deliver oxygen at higher levels than a nasal cannula.
- Incentive Spirometer
    - Handheld plastic contraption used after surgery to encourage deep breathing.
- Nasal cannula
    - Tubing with prongs for nostrils connected to Oxygen canister.

- Nebulizer
    - Aerosolizes liquid medications for inhalation
    - Mask worn over face (similar to oxygen face mask) connected to small (sometimes handheld) machine.

- Oxygen
    - Cannister and regulator found at the base of all hospital beds

- Suction
    - Tubing connected to vacuum container, used to suck liquids (spit, blood, etc.) from character's mouth to clear airway.

- Ventilator
    - Machine that breathes for a patient unable to breathe for themselves
    - Consists of ventilator machine with screen displaying rate, depth, and pressure of breaths, a humidifier, plastic tubing connected to ET tube secured to the patient's face.
    - Makes regular whooshing sounds and several different kinds of beeps.

SURGERY

- Anesthesia machine
    - Large, wheeled cart with drawers, computer screen, plastic tubing, and gas canisters, located at the head of the surgical table.
    - Anesthesiologist will be sitting beside it.

- Clamps (Locking Forceps)
    - Scissor-like instrument used to clamp tissue together

- Drapes
    - Blue paper sheets draped over patient to maintain sterile field

- Electrosurgical unit ("Bovie")
    - Pen-sized instrument used to cauterize small blood vessels

- Forceps
    - Tweezer-like instrument used for grasping.

- Hemostat
    - A commonly used clamp.

- Laparoscopic instruments
    - Metal rod with camera that is inserted into patient's body through a small incision. Camera projects visual to tv screen, allowing surgeon to operate without making a large incision.

- Procedure light (surgical light)
    - Bright light over surgical table.
    - Handles covered in plastic

- Retractors
    - Heavy silver instruments used to hold back flesh.
    - Often the medical student's job is to hold retractors.

- Scalpel
    - Sharp blade used to cut through skin and tissue.

- Surgical Gown
    - Sterile, blue paper gown worn over scrubs in the OR
    - Must be donned appropriately after scrubbing in.

- Surgical Gloves
    - White or pale brown sterile gloves.
    - Must be donned appropriately after scrubbing in.

- Sutures
    - Medical term for stitches.
    - White sterile thread connected to thin, curved needle.

URINARY

- Foley catheter ("Foley")
    - Plastic tubing placed up urethra to drain the bladder.
    - Stays in place (indwelling catheter)
    - Drains into a plastic bag at the foot of the bed.

- Straight catheter ("Straight Cath")
    - Straight plastic tubing used to drain the bladder
    - One-time use (intermittent catheterization)

APPENDIX 3: MEDICAL LEXICON

PROFESSIONAL ARGOT

- Admit = Bring patient into the hospital, ward, or unit.

- A&Ox4 = Alert and Oriented to person, place, time, and reason.

- AMA = Against Medical Advice

- Aspirate = To suck in
    - To unintentionally breathe something in
    - To draw out fluid or tissue through a needle

- Attending = a board-certified doctor who has completed their training.

- Consent = to obtain informed consent from a patient.

- Chief complaint = why the patient came to the hospital or clinic.
    - Discharge ("DC") = to release to home or care facility

- Dispo = Disposition. Where the patient goes after the hospital.

- DNR = Do not Resuscitate

- Drop = to insert
    - To "drop a line" means to start an IV

- Found down = found without a pulse
    - If someone was "found down" providers do not know how long they have been pulseless, so CPR should not be initiated.

- Grand Rounds: Teaching conference held monthly.

- GSW = Gunshot wound

- H&P = History and Physical
- HPI = History of Present Illness
- House = the hospital
- -ID = number of times per day
    - BID = twice daily
    - TID = three-times daily
    - QID = (you guessed it!) four times daily
    - QD = once daily
    - QHS = once at night.
- In-house: Physically at the hospital and available
- IM = intramuscular (into the muscle)
- IV = intravenous (into the veins)
- Is&Os = Ins and Outs
    - What patient has eaten/drank vs. what they have eliminated.
- Lytes = electrolytes
    - "Check lytes" means to get a BMP
- M&M: Morbidity and Mortality conference
    - Dreaded conference where physicians discuss cases that went wrong.
    - Slang: D&D = Death and Donuts.
- Rounds: When the medical team sees their patients
    - Prerounding: When medical students and residents see their patients before rounds, often during the very early hours of the morning.
- NPO = *Nil per os*: Nothing by mouth
- Pass-down = A meeting at the change of shift where the outgoing team relays all pertinent medical information to the incoming team.
- PMH (Past Medical History) = a list of all the patient's illnesses, injuries, and surgeries.
- PO = *per os:* By mouth

- PRN = *Pro re nata:* As Needed
- Push = to give medications by IV
- ROS (Review of Systems) = A physician's overview of organ systems not related to the patient's chief complaint.
- SOAP note: progress note written by a doctor.
- Sterile field: the area during a surgery that is kept completely sterile.
- Tap = use a needle to withdraw fluid from a body cavity
    o Spinal tap, peritoneal/abdominal tap (also called paracentesis)
- Tib/Fib = Tibia and fibula
- Tox-screen: Toxicology screen for legal and illegal drugs.
- WNL = Within Normal Limits

> The saying is that WNL actually stands for "we never looked."

SLANG

- Ambo/Ambu = Ambulance
- Ambu bag = BVM
- Anxious female = nothing is actually wrong with her
    o Often used for female patients when doctors can't figure out what's wrong.
- B52 = cocktail of medications used to make a violent or out-of-control patient sleepy
    o More formally called "chemical restraint"
- Banana Bag = IV hangover relief
    o Got its name from its yellow color.
- Bounce = to refuse an admission
- Bounce back = to return to the hospital (or the floor) shortly after discharge or transfer
- Bordie = someone with borderline personality disorder

- o Often used for patients who are manipulative and dramatic

- Bread & Butter = the basics
- Bucking the Vent = A patient fighting against the ventilator
- Cath = to catheterize a patient.
- Chocolate hostage = constipated patient
- Chemical restraint = use of sedatives to calm an aggressive or overactive patient.
- Chronic pain = drug seeker
- Circling the drain = very close to death
- Coke stroke = stroke caused by cocaine use.
- Consented = patient has given informed consent
- Covacation = when a provider gets 2 weeks paid leave after testing positive for COVID.
- Cracking the chest = an open thoracotomy, a surgical procedure requiring sawing through ribs to access the chest cavity.
- Crumping = getting sicker quickly
- Darwin award = someone who died doing something stupid
- Death sh*ts = watery diarrhea that occurs shortly after death
- Drug seeker = patient coming to clinic/ED for the express purpose of getting more of whatever drug they're addicted to.
- Dump = to transfer a complicated patient to another service to get out of having to care for them
- Elope = when a patient leaves the hospital AMA and without telling anyone.
- Frequent Flyer = someone who visits ED regularly
- High risk = the patient has HIV or hepatitis, so be extra careful.
- House = Hospital
  - o In-house = in the hospital and on-service
- Idiot-pathic = idiot doctor gave up on trying to find the cause

> **Idiopathic** means unknown cause. **Idiotpathic** means an idiot doctor just couldn't figure it out!

- Lead Poisoning = gunshot wound
    - Several iterations: Acute Lead Poisoning, High-Velocity Lead Poisoning, etc.

- Line = IV line

- NPS = New Parent Syndrome

- One point restraint = urinary catheter that keeps a patient from moving around too much.

- Pimping = the attending asking rapid-fire questions of medical student or intern.

- Rig = Ambulance

- Roid Rage = Propensity for patients on high doses of steroids to lose their sh*t.

- Rolled back = patient is rolled (in a gurney or hospital bed) to the operating area.

- Scut = menial work given to interns and med students
    - Ranges from combing through old charts to getting the team coffee.

- Snowed = patient who is sleepy due to medications
    - Can be used as an adjective or verb: "the psychiatrist snowed the patient."

- Snorkel = breathing tube

- Soft blood pressure = blood pressure that is on the low end of normal

- Trainwreck = patient with lots of health problems.

- Turf = foisting a patient (usually a complicated one) on another team without solid medical justification.

- Turf war = when a patient gets referred back and forth between different teams in the hospital because no one wants to care for them.

- TVGT = Patient who has the trifecta: a Trach, a Vent, and a G-Tube

- Worried Well = anxious patient that has nothing wrong with them

- Whale = obese or morbidly obese patient

- Whale Tarp = bariatric sling to transfer obese patients.
    - Used by nurses and surgeons in OR

- Vegetable = patient on a ventilator with minimal brain function
    - Veggie Garden = Neuro ICU (where ventilated patients are cared for)

- Vet check = nonverbal patient brought to ER without someone to tell the providers what is wrong.

- Virgin abdomen = patient who has never had abdominal surgery.

- Vitamin H = Haldol
    - An antipsychotic medication often used to 'snow' a patient.

- Zebras = rare medical conditions
    - Comes from the saying "when you hear hoofbeats think horses, not zebras."

Please note the racist, ableist, and sexist overtones of some of this slang. Doctors and nurses are people, subject to all the whims and failings of everyone else. My goal with this book is to present the medical profession as it is—warts and all. After all, warts make for interesting characters. But before you slap on a wart, make sure you're doing it for the right reason.

GLOSSARY

A

- **Abdomen:** Anatomic term for the belly area.
- **Abdominal:** Relating to the abdomen.
- **Abrasion:** A wound where the skin has been scraped away
- **ACA:** The Affordable Care Act – also known as "Obamacare"
- **ACLS:** Advanced Cardiac Life Support
- **ADLs:** Activities of Daily Living, such as dressing, eating, and bathing.
- **ADD/ADHD:** Attention Deficit Disorder/Attention Deficit Hyperactivity Disorder.
- **AED:** Automated External Defibrillator
- **Amiodarone:** Medication used to treat potentially fatal heart rhythms.
- **Anaphylaxis:** Dangerous allergic reaction causing hives and throat swelling
- **Antivenom:** Treatment for venomous snakebites.
- **APP:** Advanced Practice Provider
- **Artery:** A large blood vessel leading away from the heart
- **Aspirate:** To inhale material into the lungs.
- **Asymptomatic:** No symptoms
- **Asystole:** No electrical activity of the heart (flat-lining)
- **Ativan (Lorazepam):** Benzodiazepine medication used to treat anxiety
- **ATP:** The energy unit of all cells.
- **Atropine:** Medication used to treat slow heart rate

B

- **Backboard:** Rigid plastic board used to transport injured patients.
- **Bag Valve Mask (BVM):** Rigid plastic balloon that attaches to face mask, used to force air into lungs during CPR.
- **Bair hugger:** Plastic blanket filled with warm air, used to keep patients warm during surgery.
- **BIPOC:** Black, Indigenous, People of Color
- **Black Widow:** Venomous spider that causes severe high blood pressure.
- **Blood glucose:** Blood sugar
- **Blood pressure (BP):** The force of blood against the walls of the arteries.
- **BLS:** Basic Life Support
- **Bovie:** Surgical instrument used to electrically cauterize blood vessels.
- **Bradycardia:** A slow heart rate
- **Bradypnea:** A slow breathing rate
- **Brown Recluse:** Venomous spider whose bites cause painful, ulcerating lesions.
- **CABG:** Coronary Artery Bypass Grafting (open heart surgery).

C

- **Cadaver:** Dead body
- **Carotid artery:** The large artery in the neck (where you take your pulse)
- **Census:** How many patients a provider is responsible for caring for at any given time.
- **Cervical Collar (C-Collar):** Rigid plastic collar used to immobilize the neck and prevent vertebral fragments from severing the spinal cord.
- **Cervical Spine (C-spine):** The 7 vertebrae in the neck.
- **Clostridium dificile (C. diff):** Contagious bacteria notorious for causing malodorous diarrhea.
- **Chest compressions (compressions):** Pressing on the chest during CPR.

- **Chest tube:** Thin plastic tube inserted in the chest to remove fluid or air from the thorax.
- **Clouded:** A state of mildly impaired consciousness or fogginess.
- **CNA:** Certified Nursing Assistant
- **CNM:** Certified Nurse Midwife
- **CNS:** Central nervous system—the brain and spinal cord.
- **Code blue (Code):** Code called on the hospital overhead system if someone's heart stops beating.
- **Code team:** The medical team responsible for responding to Code Blues.
- **Colostomy:** Surgical opening connecting the colon to an external containment device (colostomy bag).
- **Coma:** A state of complete unconsciousness, characterized by lack of responsiveness to any stimuli.
- **Comatose:** The state of being in a coma.
- **Contusion:** A bruise
- **Convulsions:** Uncontrolled muscle contractions that cause violent shaking of the limbs.
- **COVID:** Coronavirus-19
- **COW/WOW:** Computer on Wheels/Workstation on Wheels
- **CPR:** Cardiopulmonary Resuscitation
- **Cricothyrotomy:** Emergency procedure used to establish an airway by cutting through the front of the neck and into the windpipe.
- **CRNA:** Certified Registered Nurse Anesthetist
- **CT Scan**: Computed Tomography Scan.

D

- **Defibrillation:** Providing an electric shock to try and return the heart to its normal rhythm
- **Dehydration:** A negative fluid balance. Can be caused by inadequate water intake or by fluid losses.

- **Dialysis:** Treatment that removes toxins and waste products from the blood. Used for patients with severe kidney disease.

- **Diaphragm:** The muscle that controls breathing.

- **Differential Diagnosis:** A list of possible disorders that could be causing symptoms, ranked from most likely (or most dangerous) to least likely.

- **DKA:** Diabetic Ketoacidosis. A high blood sugar crisis.

- **Deep Vein Thrombosis (DVT):** A blood clot in the veins, usually found in the veins of the calf.

- **DNP:** Doctor of Nursing Practice. Doctoral level nursing degree.

- **DNR:** Do Not Resuscitate

- **DO:** Doctor of Osteopathy (equivalent to an MD)

- **Drowning:** Death by suffocation due to submersion in liquid.

E

- **ECT:** Electroconvulsive Therapy.

- **Electrocardiogram/Electrokardiogram (ECG/EKG):** Test to look at the electrical rhythms of the heart

- **Electroencephalogram (EEG):** Test to look at the electrical pattern of the brain

- **Electrolytes:** Chemicals in the blood, such as sodium and potassium, which are used to maintain many cellular processes.

- **Endotracheal tube (ET tube):** Thin plastic tube used for intubation.

- **EMT:** Emergency Medical Technician

- **Extracorporeal Membrane Oxygenation (ECMO):** Machine that oxygenates blood outside the body, similar to a heart-lung machine.

- **Extubate:** The process of pulling out the endotracheal tube.

F

- **Femoral artery:** The large artery in the groin.

- **Femur:** The thigh bone. Longest and thickest bone in the body.

- **Fibula:** The thin, delicate bone of the lower leg.
- **Foley:** A plastic tube inserted into the urethra and left in place to drain the bladder.
- **Forceps:** Surgical instrument used for grasping small objects.
- **Fracture:** A broken bone
- **Frostbite:** When water in skin tissue freezes due to cold exposure. Can be superficial or deep.
- **Frostnip:** Redness of skin due to cold exposure.

G

- **G-tube:** Feeding tube surgically inserted through the abdomen.
- **GI:** Gastrointestinal
- **Glucose:** A simple sugar. Necessary for all cellular processes.
- **GSW:** Gunshot wound
- **Gurney:** Narrow, wheeled bed with rails and adjustable height.

H

- **H&P:** History and Physical
- **Haldol:** Potent antipsychotic medication
- **Heat Exhaustion:** Fatigue, headache, nausea/vomiting, dizziness, and profuse sweating, caused by heat. Often exacerbated by exertion. Generally not life-threatening.
- **Heat Stroke:** Life-threatening heat emergency characterized by hyperthermia and changes in mental status.
- **Heimlich Maneuver:** A maneuver used to dislodge a foreign body from the throat during choking.
- **Hematoma:** Pooled blood
- **Hemorrhage:** Profuse blood loss
- **Hemostat:** Surgical tool used to control bleeding. Looks like blunt scissors.

- **Herniate:** When part of an organ is pushed out of its normal body cavity through a small hole.

- **High Altitude** Cerebral Edema (HACE): Fluid on the brain caused by high altitude.
    - Also called Acute Mountain Sickness.

- **High Altitude Pulmonary Edema (HAPE):** Fluid on the lungs caused by altitude.

- **Brain herniation:** The brain is forced out of the skull and through the hole leading down into the spinal cord. Fatal if not reversed immediately.

- **HIPAA:** Health Insurance Portability and Accountability Act

- **Hospitalist:** Doctor who primarily cares for patients in the hospital

- **House:** The hospital

- **Humerus:** The bone of the upper arm.

- **Hypertension:** High blood pressure

- **Hyperthermia:** Elevated body temperature (>104°F)

- **Hypotension:** Low blood pressure.

- **Hypothermia:** Low body temperature (<95°F)

- **Hypovolemic:** Low volume of blood.

I

- **Inflatable Pneumatic Device (IPC):** Inflatable cuffs worn around the calves used to prevent blood clots in hospitalized patients

- **ICI:** Intracardiac injection – an injection straight into the heart

- **ICP:** Intracranial Pressure – the pressure of fluids on the brain inside the skull.

- **Intubate:** Procedure to thread a thin plastic tube (endotracheal tube) into the lungs, allowing for external ventilation (i.e., from a BVM or a ventilator)

- **IM:** Intramuscular (into the muscle)

- **IV:** Intravenous (into the veins)

L

- **Laceration:** A cut, often with irregular or torn edges.
- **Lethargic:** A mildly decreased state of consciousness, with diminished and/or slowed response to the environment.
- **LGBTQ+:** Lesbian, Gay, Bisexual, Transexual, Queer, and more.
- **Log roll:** A technique used to maintain C-spine while rolling a patient onto their side.

M

- **Malnutrition:** Inadequate intake or insufficient absorption of calories, vitamins, and nutrients.
- **Maxillofacial surgeon:** Dentist specialized in surgical reconstruction of the face and jaw.
- **MCS:** Minimally Conscious State
- **MD:** Medical Doctorate
- **MRI:** Magnetic Resonance Imaging
- **Myocardial Infarction:** The medical term for a heart attack.

N

- **Naloxone (Narcan):** A medication used to treat opioid overdose.
- **Nasal cannula:** Plastic tubing the delivers oxygen to the nose
- **Nasogastric Tube (NG tube):** Plastic tube threaded down a nostril into the stomach.
- **Necrotic:** Dead or dying tissue.
- **Neurodivergent:** Someone whose brains work in a way that isn't typical, such as people with Autism or ADHD.
- **Neuron:** A type of cell that uses electricity to send and receive signals within the brain and spinal cord.
- **Nerve:** A type of cell that uses electricity to transmit signals between the brain/spinal cord and the rest of the body.

- **Nitroglycerin:** Medication used to relieve pain and increase blood flow to the heart during a myocardial infarction (heart attack).
- **Normotensive:** Normal blood pressure.
- **NP:** Nurse Practitioner
- **NPO:** *nil per os.* Nothing by mouth.

O

- **Obstetrician-Gynecologist:** A doctor specialized in treating the female reproductive system, including pregnancy and fertility.
- **Obtunded:** A severely decreased state of consciousness, with diminished and/or slowed response to the environment.
- **Oliguria:** Low urine production
- **OR:** Operating Room
- **OT:** Occupational Therapy/Therapist

P

- **PA:** Physician Assistant
- **Palpitations:** A feeling that the heart is galloping or beating unevenly.
- **Pap smear:** Screening test for cervical cancer
- **Pathognomonic:** Characteristic of a particular disease, injury, or condition.
- **PEA:** Pulseless Electrical Activity, meaning the heart's electricity is not generating a heartbeat.
- **Pediatrician:** A doctor specialized in caring for children.
- **Pericardium:** The fibrous sac that surrounds the heart
- **PNS:** Peripheral nervous system—the nerves.
- **PEG tube:** Percutaneous Endoscopic Gastrostomy. Feeding tube surgically inserted through abdomen.
- **Petechiae:** Red/purple spots on skin caused by burst blood vessels.
- **PET Scan:** Positron Emission Tomography Scan.

- **PHI:** Protected Health Information
- **Physiatrist:** Doctor specializing in patients needing physical rehabilitation.
- **Piloerection:** Goosebumps
- **PPE:** Personal Protective Equipment, such as gloves, face masks, and gowns.
- **Prognosis:** The likely outcome of a disease, injury, or condition.
- **Prolonged Mechanical Ventilation (PVM):** Needing to consistently be on a ventilator for more than three weeks.
- **Prone:** Lying face down.
- **Proned/Proning:** Placing a patient who is having trouble breathing in a face-down position to increase lung capacity
- **Psychiatrist:** Medical doctor (MD or DO) specialized in the treatment of mental illness
- **Psychologist:** Mental health providers (Master's or Ph.D. in Psychology) trained in psychotherapy and psychoanalysis.
- **PT:** Physical Therapy/Therapist
- **PTSD:** Post-Traumatic Stress Disorder
- **Pulse oximeter:** Device used to measure blood oxygen levels
- **PVS:** Persistent Vegetative State

Q

- **QRS Complex:** The typical EKG heart rhythm pattern.

R

- **Radial artery:** The large artery in the wrist.
- **Radius:** The large bone in the lower arm.
- **RBCs:** Red Blood Cells
- **Refeeding Syndrome:** A dangerous syndrome characterized by a shift in electrolytes caused by reintroduction of food after a period of starvation.
- **Refractory Status Epilepticus (RSE):** Aseizure lasting more than 5 minutes that does not respond to medication. Indication for a therapeutic coma.

- **Rhythm Strip:** The result of an EKG: the heart's electrical rhythm, printed on white paper with red lines.
- **Rigors:** Chills and shaking during a fever
- **Rigor mortis:** The stiffness of death
- **Rounding:** The process of going around the hospital to check in on every patient
- **RT:** Respiratory Therapist

S

- **Scalpel:** Sharp surgical instrument used to cut tissue
- **Scrubs:** Loose medical clothing, often light green or pale blue, worn to protect the wearer against bodily fluids and minimize transmission of contaminants.
- **Seizure:** Electrical disturbance in the brain that may or may not cause convulsions.
- **Serum sickness:** Immune reaction to venom of snakes, spiders, etc.
- **Signs:** The objective indications of disease, illness, or injury (i.e., low blood pressure)
- **Skilled Nursing Facility (SNF):** Care facility providing high-level nursing care.
- **SLP:** Speech-language Pathologist
- **Spleen:** An easily injured organ in the abdomen responsible for producing infection-fighting white blood cells (WBCs) and filtering the blood.
- **Sputum:** The stuff you cough up (phlegm)
- **Starvation:** A severe calorie deficiency. Has several stages.
- **Status epilepticus:** A seizure lasting more than 5 minutes
- **Stethoscope:** Instrument used to listen to the heart, lungs, and abdomen.
- **STI:** Sexually Transmitted Infection (previously called STDs)
- **Straight Catheter (Straight Cath):** A plastic tube inserted into the urethra to drain the bladder, then immediately removed.

> Since not all infections lead to disease, STI is more accurate than STD.

- ***Staphylococcus*:** Class of bacteria notorious for causing abscesses and wound infections.
- ***Streptococcus:*** Class of bacteria also known for causing abscesses and wound infections.
- **Stretcher:** Narrow, wheeled bed with collapsible legs. Used in the field.
- **Stupor:** Severely diminished consciousness; only minimally responsive to the environment.
- **Subconjunctival Hemorrhage:** Burst blood vessel in the eye.
- **Supine:** Lying face up.
- **Surgical Drain:** Plastic tubing, often connected to suction or suction bulb, meant to remove fluids or gas from the body.
- **Sutures:** Stitches.
- **Symptoms:** The subjective feelings of disease, illness, or injury (i.e., a stomachache)

T

- **Tachycardia:** A fast heart rate.
- **Tachypnea:** A fast breathing rate.
- **TBI:** Traumatic Brain Injury
- **TED hose:** Compression stockings designed to prevent blood clots
- **Telemetry:** In-hospital constant monitoring of heart rhythm and vitals
- **Thorax:** Anatomic term for the chest.
- **Thoracic:** Relating to the thorax.
- **Tibia:** The large bone of the lower leg.
- **Tracheostomy:** A surgical opening in the front of the neck used for patients requiring persistent ventilation.
- **Trauma shears:** Heavy-duty scissors for cutting the clothes off victims.
- **TTX:** Tetrodotoxin. A potent toxin found in pufferfish.
- **Type and screen:** Blood test to determine blood type

U

- **Ulna:** The thin, delicate bone in the lower arm.
- **Ultrasound:** Imaging study using soundwaves to generate a moving picture.
- **Urethra:** The anatomical tube leading from the bladder to the outside of the body.
- **Urologist:** A doctor specialized in the treatment of the bladder, urethra, testis, and certain kidney disorders.

V

- **Vein:** A blood vessel that returns blood to the heart.
- **Ventilate:** To force air into the lungs. Can be done manually (with BVM or mouth-to-mouth) or with ventilator.
- **Ventricular Fibrillation:** Potentially deadly heart rhythm
- **Vital Signs:** Heart rate, breathing rate, blood pressure, and temperature. Weight and blood oxygenation also sometimes included.

W

- **WBCs:** White blood cells

X

- **X-ray:** Study that uses radiation to generate a 2D image.
- **Xanax (Alprazolam):** Benzodiazepine medication used to treat anxiety.

INDEX

A

ABCDEs, *see also c-ABCs,* 46, 90-94

Abrasion, 16

Abuse, 111-122

    Adult Abuse, 119-120

    Approach to victims of, 112-113

    Child, *see also Child Abuse,* 114-116

    Domestic, *see Intimate Partner Violence,* 117-118

    Elder, *see Adult Abuse,* 119-120

    Follow-up for, 120-121

    Mandatory reporters of, 111-112

    Perpetrator red flags, 114

    Sexual, *see Sexual Assault,* 118-119

    Spousal, *see Intimate Partner Violence,* 117-118

    Victim red flags, 113-114

Addiction, 123-141

    Alcohol, 125-129

    Opioid, 129-132

Advanced Cardiac Life Support (ACLS), 105-107, 179

Advanced Practice Providers (APPS), *see also Physician Assistant and Nurse Practitioner,* 70-74

    Character sheet, 70

Airway, 90-91

    Equipment, 211

    In ACLS, 106

    Management, 90-91

    With C-spine protection, 90-91
Alcohol, 125-129
    Addiction, 126
    Alcoholic Hallucinosis, 128
    Binge drinking, 126
    Delirium Tremens (DTs), 128
    Misuse, 126
    Overdose, 126-127
    Relapse prevention, -128-129
    Use Disorder, 128
    Withdrawal, 127-128
    Withdrawal seizures, 128
Alcoholism, 126
Algor mortis, 184
Altitude Sickness, 139, 146-148
    Acute Mountain Sickness, 147
    High-Altitude Cerebral Edema, 147
    High-Altitude Pulmonary Edema, 147
Ambulance, 45-46
    Driving the, 76
    Sensory descriptors, 45
Amphetamines, *see Stimulants,* 138
Anesthesia,
    Gas machine, 21
    Post-Anesthesia Care Unit (PACU), 23-24
Anesthesiologist, 20, 22, 63
    Nurse anesthetists (CRNA), 72
Attending, 28
Automatic External Defibrillator (AED), 104-105
Autopsy, *see Post-Mortem exam,* 183-184
Avulsion injuries, 16

B

Barbiturates, *see also Sedatives,* 135-138

Bites, 142-144
    Bat, 143
    Cat, 142
    Dog, 143
    Human, 115, 117
    Snake, 143-144
    Spider, 144
Brain herniation, 163
Brainstem reflexes, 180
Benzodiazepines, *see also Sedatives,* 135-138
Blood loss, *see also Hemorrhagic Shock,* 98-99
Blood transfusion, 99
Blunt trauma, 16
Botulism, 196-197
Brain death, 180-182
Brain injury, 162, 194
    Medically induced coma due to, 164-165
Breathing, 91-92
    Rate, 36
    Trial *see also Spontaneous Breathing Trial (SBT),* 174
Broken bones, *see also Fractures,* 17
Bullet wounds, 190

C

c-ABCs, *see also ABCs,* 46, 90-94
C-spine, 90-91
    Protection, 91
C-collar, 91
Cannabis, 132-133
    Intoxication, 133
    Overdose, 133
    Types, 132
    Withdrawal, 133
Cat bite, 142

Catatonia, 198-199

Certified Nursing Assistant (CNA), *see also Nurse's Aide*, 27, 49

Certified Nurse Midwife (CNM), 72-73

Certified Registered Nurse Anesthetist (CRNA), 72

Child Abuse, 114-116
- Behavioral/Emotional signs of, 116
- Parental risk factors for, 116
- Physical signs of, 115

Chronic illness, 197-198

Circulation, 46, 92-93
- Disorders of, 92-93
- Return of spontaneous circulation (ROSC), 110

Clichés,
- Angel Nurse, 68
- Awakening, 170
- B*tch Nurse, 69
- Code Blue, 35
- Date Rape Drugs, 140-141
- Dr. Badboy, 62-63
- Emotional Shock, 100-101
- Flat-lining, 108-109
- Frequent Flyer, 12-13
- Handmaiden, 67
- HIPAA Hurdle, 30-31
- House Calls, 42-43
- Human bites, 156-157
- Kiss of Life, 157-158
- Last Words, 185-186
- Lone Wolf, 94-95
- Medically Induced Coma, 169
- Murse, 69
- Naughty Nurse, 67-68
- Only Men are Abusers, 121-122

    Physician's Assistant, 73-74

    Psychological Trauma, 17-18

    Real Doctor, 62

    Shot to the Heart, 109

    Super-Doc, 85-86

    'Tis but a Scratch, 101

    Ventilator = Coma, 178

    Visiting the Morgue, 53-54

    Watching Surgery, 24

    We Cheat Death, 78-79

Clinical Nurse Specialist (CNS), 72

Cocaine, *see also Stimulants,* 139

Contusion, 16

Consciousness, 159-160

Consult, 12, 28

Coma, 161-167

    Causes of, 162-163

    Glasgow Coma Scale, 160-161

    Monitoring, 165-166

    Outcomes, 167

    Recovery, 166-167

    Therapeutic, 164-165

Counselor, 80-81

COVID,

    Autopsies due to, 183

    Isolation units, 204

    Nursing homes, 50

    Personal protective equipment, 12

    Ventilators, 172

    Visitation during, 29

CPR, *see also Cardiopulmonary Resuscitation,* 102-104

    Dos and Don'ts, 103

    Indications, 102

    Performing, 103
CT scan, 41

D

Date rape drugs, 140-141

Death, 177-185
    Brain, 180-182
    Cardiopulmonary, 179-180
    Pronouncing, 182-183
    Rattle, 179
    Stages, 184-185
    Timing of, 185
    Types, 179-182

Decisionmakers, Medical, 31, 161

Dehydration, 153

Diagnosis, differential, 60

Digoxin, 196

Disability, 93-94
    After coma, 167
    In ABCDEs, 93-94
    In chronic illness, 197-198

Dislocation, 16

Doctor, *see also Physicians,* 57-64
    Corrupt, 199-200

Dog bite, 143

Domestic Violence, *see also Intimate Partner Violence,* 117-118

Do Not Resuscitate Order (DNR), 107-108

Drowning, 148-150
    Chance of survival by duration of submersion, 149
    Dry, 147

Dying,
    Signs and Symptoms, 177-179

E

ECMO (Extracorporeal Membrane Oxygenation), 32

EEG (Electroencephalogram), 32, 164
    In diagnosis of brain death, 181

Elder abuse, *see also Adult Abuse* 119-120

Emergency, Approach to, 89-95

Emergency Department (ED), 9-13
    Sensory Descriptors, 10
    Setting, 11
    Team, 11-12
    Triage, 9

Emergency Medical Responders, *see also First Responders*, 76

Emergency Medical Service (EMS) Providers, 75-79
    Character sheet, 75
    Day in the life, 78

Emergency Medical Technician (EMT), 76-77

ER Doctor, *see also ED doctor,* 12

Evidence collection kit, *see also Rape Kit,* 119

Exposure, 94

Extubation, 174

F

Fellow, 27-28

First Responders, *see also Emergency Medical Responders,* 76

Fluid resuscitation, 99

Fractures, 17

Frostbite, 151-152

G

Glasgow Coma Scale, 160-161

Gunshot wounds, 16, 194

H

Hallucinogens, 133-135
    Types, 133
    Intoxication, 134-135
    Withdrawal, 135

Healthcare System, 201-202
    Medicare, 201
    Medicaid, 201
Health Insurance, 201-202
    Marketplace, 202
Heat Exhaustion, 145
Heat Stroke, 145-146
HIPAA (Health Insurance Portability & Accountability Act), 30
History and Physical (H&P), 59
Hospice, *see also Palliative Care*, 50-51
    Hospice House, 51
Hospital 25-30
    Food, 29
    Rooms, 25-27
    Sensory, 26
    Team, 27
    Visiting the, 29-30
Hospitalist, 27
Human bites, 115, 156-157
Hypothermia, 150-151
    Therapeutic, 162

I

Imaging Center, 40-42
    Sensory descriptors, 40
Injuries
    After getting beaten up, 191-192
    Characteristic of adult abuse, 119-120
    Characteristic of child abuse, 115
    Characteristic of intimate partner violence, 117-118
    Having sex after, 195-196
    Recovery times for, 192-195
Inpatient Team, 27
Intensive Care Unit (ICU), 32-

    Sensory Descriptors, 33-35
    Setting, 32-24
    Team, 34-35
Intern, 28
Intimate Partner Violence, 117-118
    Characteristic injuries, 117-118
Intubation, 91, 172

K

Kwashiorkor, 155

L

Lab, 39-40
    Sensory descriptors, 39
Lacerations, 189-190
Lazarus Sign, 181
Livor mortis, 185
LSD, 133-134

M

Malnutrition, 156
Marasmus, 155
Marijuana, *see Cannabis*, 132-133
Medical Equipment (Appendix 2), 205-214
Medical Lexicon (Appendix 3), 215-20
    Professional argot, 215-217
    Slang, 217-220
Medical Student, 57
Medically Induced Coma, *see also Therapeutic Coma*, 164-165
Minimally Conscious State, 169
Morgue, 52-54
    Sensory descriptors, 52
    Team, 52-53
Morticians, 53
Mortuary, 53

MRI, 41-42

N

Naloxone, 131
Narcan, 131
Neurological Exam, 166
Neurologist, 64, 165
Nurse, 65-69
    Character sheet, 65-66
    Clichés, 67-69
    Day in the life, 66-67
    Role, 66
Nurse Practitioner (NP), 72
Nurse's Aide, *see also CNA*, 27, 49
Nursing Facility, 48-50

O

O-negative blood, 99
Occupational Therapist (OT), 43, 81
Operating room (OR), 21-23
    Atmosphere, 22
    Scrubbing into, 22
    Sensory descriptors, 21
    Staff, 22
    Surgical Tools, 22-23
Opioids, 129-132, 141
    Intoxication, 130
    Epidemic, 141
    Overdose, 130-131
    Relapse prevention, 131-132
    Types, 129-130
    Withdrawal 130-131
Organ donation, 181
Outpatient Clinic, 36-39
    Sensory Details, 37

Specialties, 38-39

Team, 36-37

P

Painful stimuli, 89

Palliative Care, 43, 50-51

    Locations, 51

    Team, 50-51

Pallor mortis,184

Paramedic, 77

Parts of a Hospital (Appendix 1), 203-204

Pathologist, 52, 64

    Forensic, 52

Patient

    Sitter, 82

    Transport, 82

Penetrating trauma, 16

Persistent Vegetative State (PVS), 167-169

PET scan, 42

Pharmacist, 82-82

Phencyclidine, (PCP), 133-135

Physiatrist, 15

Physical Therapist (PT), 83

Physician, *see also Doctor*, 57-64

    Character sheet, 57-58

    Clichés, 62-63

    Day in the life, 60-61

    Role, 59

    Stereotypes by specialty, 63-64

    Training, 57

Physician Assistant (PA), 71-71

    Character sheet, 70

Pimping, 29

Poisoning,

    Alcohol, 126-127
    Carbon Monoxide, 162
    Honey, 196-197
    Tetrodotoxin, 196
Post-Anesthesia Care Unit (PACU), 23-24
    Sensory descriptors, 24
Post-Mortem exam, *see Autopsy*, 183-184
Posttraumatic Stress Disorder (PTSD), 19
    In ventilated patients, 173
Preliminary Survey, 17
Preoperative area, "Pre-op," 20-21
    Sensory descriptors, 20
Primary Care Practitioner (PCP), 36-37
Protected Health Information (PHI), 30
Psilocybin, 133-135

R

Rabies, 143
Rape, 118-119
    Kit, *see also Evidence Collection Kit*, 119
Refeeding Syndrome, 156
Refractory Status Epilepticus (RSE), 165
Rehabilitation hospital, 46-48
    Equipment, 47
    Sensory descriptors, 46
Rescue breathing, 103, 149
Resident, 28
Respiratory rate, *see also Breathing rate*, 97
Respiratory Therapist, RT, 12, 83-84
Resuscitation,
    Cardiopulmonary, 102-104
    Fluid, 99
Rigor Mortis, 184-185
Rounds, 29-29

S

Scrubbing in, 22

Secondary Survey, 18

Sedatives, 135-138
    Intoxication, 136
    Types, 135-136
    Overdose, 136
    Withdrawal, 136-138

Sexual Assault, 118-119

Shock, 96-101
    Cardiogenic, 100
    Distributive, *see also Neurogenic shock*, 100
    Emotional, *see also Takotsubo's Cardiomyopathy*, 100-101
    Hallmarks, 97
    Hemorrhagic, 98-99
    Hypovolemic, 98-99
    Neurogenic, *see also Distributive shock*, 100
    Septic, 100

Skilled Nursing Facility, 48-49
    Sensory descriptors, 48

Snake bite, 143-144

Social Worker, 84-85

Specialty Clinics, 38-39

Speech & Language Pathologist (SLP), 44, 84

Spider bite, 144

Spinal reflexes, 181

Sprain, 17

Spontaneous Breathing Trial (SBT), 174

Starvation, 154-155

Sterile field, 22

Sternal rub, 89

Stimulants, 138-140
    Types, 138-139

Intoxication, 139

　　Withdrawal, 140

Strangulation, 118, 162

Surgical tools, 22-23

Sutures, 193

T

Takotsubo's Cardiomyopathy, 101

Telemetry, 11

Tetrodotoxin (TTX), 196

Therapeutic Coma, 164-167, 160

　　In brain injury, 165

　　In refractory status epilepticus, 165

　　Monitoring, 165-166

　　Outcomes, 167

　　Recovery, 166-167

Therapist

　　Occupational, ,81

　　Physical, 83

　　Psychological *see also Counselor*, 80

　　Respiratory, 83-83

　　Speech, *see also Speech Language Pathologist*, 84

Therapeutic hypothermia,162

Thoracotomy, resuscitative, 18

Thorax, 99

Tourniquet, 190

Tracheostomy, 174-175

Transport, patient, 82

Trauma Center, 14-16

　　Levels of, 15-16

　　Sensory Descriptors, 14

　　Team, 15

Traumatic Injuries, 16-18

　　Approach to, 17-18

Blunt trauma, 16
  Gunshot wounds, 16
  Penetrating trauma, 16
  Types of, 16-17
  Treatment of, 17-18
Triage, 9
Type and screen, 99

U
Ultrasound, 42
Universal Donor blood type, 99

V
Ventilators, 171-176
  Experience of being ventilated, 172-173
  Weaning off, 173-174
Vital signs, 36, 96-97

W
White coats, 28, 61
Wound, 16-18
  Care, 18
  Types, 16-17

X
X-ray, 41

WORKS CITED

CHAPTER 1: EMERGENCY DEPARTMENT

1. "Emergency Medical Treatment & Labor Act (EMTALA)." *CMS*, https://www.cms.gov/Regulations-and-Guidance/Legislation/EMTALA.

2. Sava, Nicos, and Tolga Tezcan. "To Reduce Emergency Room Wait Times, Tie Them to Payments." *Harvard Business Review*, 6 Feb. 2019, https://hbr.org/2019/02/to-reduce-emergency-room-wait-times-tie-them-to-payments#:~:text=The%20average%20wait%20time%20in,an%20hour%20and%20a%20half.&text=and%202.25...-,The%20average%20hospital%20emergency%20department%20(ED)%20patient%20in%20the%20United,2.25%20hours%20before%20being%20discharged.

CHAPTER 2: TRAUMA CENTER

1. Page, David W. *Body Trauma: A Writer's Guide to Wounds and Injuries.* Behler Publications, 2007.

2. Nickson, Chris. "Resuscitative Thoracotomy." *Life in the Fast Lane • LITFL*, 3 Nov. 2020, litfl.com/resuscitative-thoracotomy/.

CHAPTER 3: SURGICAL SUITE

1. Farmer, Heather. Physician Assistant in Cardiology. Personal Interview by Natalie Dale. 7 March 2021.

2. Ollier, Ryan. Certified Registered Nurse Anesthetist. Personal Interview by Natalie Dale. 4 March 2021.

CHAPTER 4: HOSPITAL FLOORS

1. "Health Insurance Portability and Accountability Act of 1996 (HIPAA)." *Centers for Disease Control and Prevention*, Centers for Disease Control and Prevention, 14 Sept. 2018, https://www.cdc.gov/phlp/publications/topic/hipaa.html#:~:text=The%20Health%20Insurance%20Portability%20and,the%20patient's%20consent%20or%20knowledge.

CHAPTER 5: ICU

1. "ICU Outcomes." *Philip R. Lee Institute for Health Policy Studies*, University of California San Francisco, 2021, https://healthpolicy.ucsf.edu/icu-outcomes.

CHAPTER 6: CLINIC

1. "MRI Bore Sizes and Benefits." *GE Healthcare Systems*, 16 Jan. 2019, https://www.gehealthcare.com/article/mri-bore-sizes-and-benefits#:~:text=Traditionally%2C%20MRI%20scanners%20have%20had,this%2C%20many%20patients%20reported%20claustrophobia.

2. Krans, Brian. "PET Scan: Definition, Purpose, Procedure, and Results." *Healthline*, Healthline Media, 17 Sept. 2018, https://www.healthline.com/health/pet-scan#:~:text=After%20the%20test%2C%20you%20can,and%20infants%20during%20this%20time.

CHAPTER 7: OTHER SETTINGS

1. "Does Medicare Pay for Nursing Home?" *Medical News Today*, MediLexicon International, https://www.medicalnewstoday.com/articles/does-medicare-pay-for-nursing-home#which-parts-of-medicare-cover-it.

2. Crecelius, Charles. "Working to Reduce Skilled Nursing Facility Hospitalizations." *Caring for the Ages*, https://www.caringfortheages.com/article/S1526-4114(14)00007-9/pdf#:~:text=The%20most%20common%20diagnoses%20associated,acute%20renal%20failure%20(3.9%25).

3. Roe, Sam. "Misery: Inside a 1-Star Nursing Home." *Chicagotribune.com*, Chi-

cago Tribune, 30 Jan. 2019, https://www.chicagotribune.com/lifestyles/chi-nursing-homes-feb08-story.html.

4. Balko, Radley. "Opinion | It's Time to Abolish the Coroner." *The Washington Post*, WP Company, 30 Mar. 2019, https://www.washingtonpost.com/news/the-watch/wp/2017/12/12/its-time-to-abolish-the-coroner/.

5. "Death Investigations." *Last Week Tonight*, HBO, 19 May 2019, https://www.youtube.com/watch?v=hnoMsftQPY8&t=1s&ab_channel=LastWeekTonight. Accessed 24 Sept. 2021.

CHAPTER 8: PHYSICIANS

1. Levy, Sandra, and Leslie Kane. "Medscape Malpractice Report 2017." *Medscape*, 15 Nov. 2017, https://www.medscape.com/slideshow/2017-malpractice-report-6009206#1.

CHAPTER 9: NURSES

1. Dale, Karen. Certified Rehabilitation Registered Nurse. Personal Interview by Natalie Dale. 14 April 2021.

2. Vermeulen, Aletta. Registered Nurse. Personal Interview by Natalie Dale. 3 March 2021.

3. Kahsay, Woldegebriel, Gebregziabher, et al. "Sexual Harassment against Female Nurses: A Systematic Review." *BMC Nursing*, BioMed Central, 13 July 2020, https://bmcnurs.biomedcentral.com/articles/10.1186/s12912-020-00450-w.

CHAPTER 10: ADVANCED PRACTICE PROVIDERS

1. Farmer, Heather. Physician Assistant in Cardiology. Personal Interview by Natalie Dale. 7 March 2021.

2. Ollier, Ryan. Certified Registered Nurse Anesthetist. Personal Interview by Natalie Dale. 4 March 2021.

3. "What Is a CNS?" *NACNS: National Association of Clinical Nurse Specialists*, 21 Oct. 2021, https://nacns.org/about-us/what-is-a-cns/.

CHAPTER 11: EMS PROVIDERS

1. "Office of Emergency Medical Services." *EMT Scope of Practice*, West Virginia Health and Human Services, 30 Jan. 2021, https://www.wvoems.org/medical-direction/scope-of-practice/emt-scope-of-practice.

2. "National EMS Scope of Practice Model." *Paramedic Scope of Practice*, National Highway Traffic Safety Association, Feb. 2007, https://www.ems.gov/pdf/education/EMS-Education-for-the-Future-A-Systems-Approach/National_EMS_Scope_Practice_Model.pdf.

3. "What's the Difference between an EMT and a Paramedic?" *UCLA CPC*, 2 Sept. 2021, https://www.cpc.mednet.ucla.edu/node/27.

CHAPTER 12: OTHER HEALTHCARE PERSONNEL

1. Vermeulen, Janettha. Physical Therapist. Personal Interview. By Natalie Dale. 28 Feb 2021.

2. McCarthy, Amy. Social Worker. Personal Interview by Natalie Dale. 20 Feb 2021.

3. Defusco, Concerts. Medical Social Worker. Personal Interview. By Natalie Dale. 8 March 2021.

4. "Ain't Nobody Got Time for That" Meme. Kimberly "Sweet Brown Wilkins" *YouTube*. 8 April 2012. https://www.youtube.com/watch?v=waEC-8GFTP4&ab_channel=NobodyGotTimeForThis.

5. O'Leary, Kevin J, et al. "How Hospitalists Spend Their Time: Insights on Efficiency and Safety." *Journal of Hospital Medicine*, U.S. National Library of Medicine, Mar. 2006, https://pubmed.ncbi.nlm.nih.gov/17219478/#:~:text=Hospitalists%20spent%2018%25%20of%20their,development%2C%20education%2C%20and%20travel.

CHAPTER 13: RESPONSE TO AN EMERGENCY

1. Seaman, Andrew M. "Be Prepared for Ambulance Wait Times." *Reuters*, Thomson Reuters, 19 July 2017, www.reuters.com/article/us-health-emergency-response-times/be-prepared-for-ambulance-wait-times-idUSKBN1A42KQ.

CHAPTER 14: SHOCK

1. Agabegi, Steven S., et al. *Step-up to Medicine*. Third ed., Wolters Kluwer, 2014.

2. "Takotsubo Cardiomyopathy (Broken-Heart Syndrome)." *Harvard Health*, 29 Jan. 2020, www.health.harvard.edu/heart-health/takotsubo-cardiomyopathy-broken-heart-syndrome.

CHAPTER 15: CPR

1. "CPR: Clean, Pretty, Reliable." *TV Tropes*, tvtropes.org/pmwiki/pmwiki.php/Main/CPRCleanPrettyReliable.

2. "Flatline." *TV Tropes*, tvtropes.org/pmwiki/pmwiki.php/Main/Flatline.

3. "Shot to the Heart." *TV Tropes*, tvtropes.org/pmwiki/pmwiki.php/Main/ShotToTheHeart.

4. Reichman, Eric F. "Chapter 37. Intracardiac Injection." *Chapter 37. Intracardiac Injection | Emergency Medicine Procedures, 2e | Access Emergency Medicine | McGraw Hill Medical*, accessemergencymedicine.mhmedical.com/content.aspx?sectionid=45343675.

5. Geocadin, Romergryko, et al. "Management of Brain Injury after Resuscitation from Cardiac Arrest." *Neurologic Clinics*, U.S. National Library of Medicine, May 2008, www.ncbi.nlm.nih.gov/pmc/articles/PMC3074242/.

6. Sandroni, Claudio, et al. "Prognostication after Cardiac Arrest." *Critical Care*, BioMed Central, 5 June 2018, ccforum.biomedcentral.com/articles/10.1186/s13054-018-2060-7#:~:text=About%2080%25%20of%20patients%20who,)%20%5B2%2C%203%5D.

CHAPTER 16: ABUSE

1. "National Child Abuse Statistics from NCA." *National Children's Alliance*, 21 Sept. 2021, https://www.nationalchildrensalliance.org/media-room/national-statistics-on-child-abuse/.

2. Scribano, Philip V., and Russell A. Faust. "Ear, Nose, and Throat Injuries in Abused Children." *Child Abuse and Neglect*, W.B. Saunders, 3 Nov. 2010, https://www.sciencedirect.com/science/article/pii/B9781416063933000373.

3. "Risk and Protective Factors Intimate Partner Violence." *Centers for Disease Control and Prevention*, Violence Prevention & Injury Center. 9 Oct. 2020, https://www.cdc.gov/violenceprevention/intimatepartnerviolence/riskprotectivefactors.html.

4. *Racial Disproportionality - Child Welfare*. Apr. 2021, https://www.childwelfare.gov/pubPDFs/racial_disproportionality.pdf.

5. Child Abuse. "Signs & Symptoms." *Child Abuse*, 2021, https://childabuse.stanford.edu/screening/signs.html.

6. Choo, Esther K, and Debra E Houry. "Managing Intimate Partner Violence in the Emergency Department." *Annals of Emergency Medicine*, U.S. National Library of Medicine, Apr. 2015, https://www.ncbi.nlm.nih.gov/pmc/articles/PMC4393790/.

7. Barkley Burnett, Lynn. "Domestic Violence Clinical Presentation: History, Physical, Causes." *Domestic Violence Clinical Presentation: History, Physical, Causes*, Medscape, 13 Oct. 2021, https://emedicine.medscape.com/article/805546-clinical#b4.

8. Curington, Molly. "The Injustice of America's Rape Kit Backlog." *The Arkansas Journal of Social Change and Public Service*, 1 Apr. 2021, https://ualr.edu/socialchange/2021/03/31/the-injustice-of-americas-rape-kit-backlog/.

9. "Preventing Elder Abuse |Violence Prevention Injury Center CDC." *Centers for Disease Control and Prevention*, Centers for Disease Control and Prevention, 2 June 2021, https://www.cdc.gov/violenceprevention/elderabuse/fastfact.html.

10. "Domestic Abuse Is a Gendered Crime." *Women's Aid*, 3 Aug. 2021, https://www.womensaid.org.uk/information-support/what-is-domestic-abuse/domestic-abuse-is-a-gendered-crime/.

11. Truman, Jennifer, and Rachel Morgan. "Nonfatal Domestic Violence 2003-2012." *Bureau of Justice Statistics: Special Report*, Apr. 2014, pp. 1–20., https://doi.org/https://bjs.ojp.gov/content/pub/pdf/ndv0312.pdf.

12. Campell, Dennis. "More than 40% of Domestic Violence Victims Are Male, Report Reveals." *The Guardian*, Guardian News and Media, 4 Sept. 2010, https://www.theguardian.com/society/2010/sep/05/men-victims-domestic-violence.

13. Published by Statista Research Department, and Jan 21. "Child Abuse in the U.S. - Perpetrators by Sex 2019." *Statista*, 21 Jan. 2021, https://www.statista.com/statistics/418470/number-of-perpetrators-in-child-abuse-cases-in-the-us-by-sex/.

14. "Violence against Trans and Non-Binary People." *VAWnet.org*, https://vawnet.org/sc/serving-trans-and-non-binary-survivors-domestic-and-sexual-violence/violence-against-trans-and.

15. Rose, Suzana. "Fact Sheet: Lesbian Partner Violence." *National Violence Against Women Prevention Research Center*, University of Missouri at St. Louis, 2000, https://mainweb-v.musc.edu/vawprevention/lesbianrx/factsheet.shtml.

16. "Get the Facts on Elder Abuse." *The National Council on Aging*, 23 Feb. 2021, https://www.ncoa.org/article/get-the-facts-on-elder-abuse.

17. "Patterns of Injury That Should Raise Suspicion for Child Abuse." *Relias Media - Continuing Medical Education Publishing*, 2005, https://www.reliasmedia.com/articles/87722-patterns-of-injury-that-should-raise-suspicion-for-child-abuse.

CHAPTER 17: DRUGS, ALCOHOL & ADDICTION

1. "10 Unusual ADDICTIONS." *Willow Springs Recovery*, www.willowspringsrecovery.com/addiction/10-unusual-addictions/.

2. "Substance-Related and Addictive Disorders." *Psychology: DSM 5*, by Saundra K. Ciccarelli and J. Noland White, 5th ed., Pearson, 2014, pp. 481–590.

3. "Alcohol Facts and Statistics." *National Institute on Alcohol Abuse and Alcoholism*, U.S. Department of Health and Human Services, June 2021, www.niaaa.nih.gov/publications/brochures-and-fact-sheets/alcohol-facts-and-statistics.

4. Zorumski, Charles F. "What Causes Alcohol-Induced Blackouts?" *Scientific American*, Scientific American, 26 Oct. 2018, https://www.scientificamerican.com/article/what-causes-alcohol-induced-blackouts/.

5. Cowen, Ethan, and Mark K Su. "Ethanol Intoxication in Adults." *UpToDate*, July 2021, www.uptodate.com/contents/ethanol-intoxication-in-adults?search=alcohol+poisoning&source=search_result&selectedTitle=1~150&usage_type=default&display_rank=1.

6. "Prescription Opioids: Overview." *Centers for Disease Control and Prevention*, Centers for Disease Control and Prevention, Mar. 2021, www.cdc.gov/drugoverdose/data/prescribing/overview.html.

7. Keating, Dan, and Samuel Grenados. "Analysis | See How Deadly Street Opioids

like 'Elephant Tranquilizer' Have Become." *The Washington Post*, WP Company, 25 Oct. 2017, www.washingtonpost.com/graphics/2017/health/opioids-scale/.

8. Cherney, Kristeen. "Coping with Opiate Withdrawal." *Healthline*, Healthline Media, 21 July 2020, www.healthline.com/health/coping-opiate-withdrawal#symptoms-andtimeline.

9. "Withdrawal Management." *Clinical Guidelines for Withdrawal Management and Treatment of Drug Dependence in Closed Settings.*, U.S. National Library of Medicine, 1 Jan. 1970, www.ncbi.nlm.nih.gov/books/NBK310652/.

10. Kaskutas, Lee Ann. "Alcoholics Anonymous Effectiveness: Faith Meets Science." *Journal of Addictive Diseases*, U.S. National Library of Medicine, 2009, www.ncbi.nlm.nih.gov/pmc/articles/PMC2746426/.

11. Swift, Robert M, and Elizabeth R Aston. "Pharmacotherapy for Alcohol Use Disorder: Current and Emerging Therapies." *Harvard Review of Psychiatry*, U.S. National Library of Medicine, 2015, www.ncbi.nlm.nih.gov/pmc/articles/PMC4790835/.

12. "Barbiturates." *DEA*, www.dea.gov/factsheets/barbiturates.

13. "Drug Street Names: The Ultimate List." *Addiction Center*, 10 Aug. 2021, www.addictioncenter.com/drugs/drug-street-names/.

14. Agabegi, Steven S., et al. *Step-up to Medicine*. Third ed., Wolters Kluwer, 2014.

15. Rahman, Abdul. "Delirium Tremens." *Stat Pearls*. U.S. National Library of Medicine, 27 Aug. 2021, https://www.ncbi.nlm.nih.gov/books/NBK482134/.

16. "Benzo Withdrawal: Timeline and Symptoms." *Medical News Today*. www.medicalnewstoday.com/articles/benzo-withdrawal#acute-withdrawal.

17. O'Connell, Ted, et al. "Gamma-Hydroxybutyrate (GHB): A Newer Drug of Abuse." *American Family Physician*, 1 Dec. 2000, www.aafp.org/afp/2000/1201/p2478.html.

18. "Opioid Rehabilitation Clinic - How Does a Methadone Clinic Work?" *American Addiction Centers*, 16 Mar. 2021, americanaddictioncenters.org/methadone-addiction/clinic-facts.

19. Assistant Secretary of Public Affairs (ASPA). "What Is the U.S. Opioid Epidemic?" *HHS.gov*, Https://Plus.google.com/+HHS, www.hhs.gov/opioids/about-the-epidemic/index.html.

20. "Opioid Overdose Crisis." *National Institute on Drug Abuse*, 1 July 2021, https://www.drugabuse.gov/drug-topics/opioids/opioid-overdose-crisis.

CHAPTER 18: ENVIRONMENTAL EMERGENCIES

1. Zane, Richard D., and Joshua M. Kosowsky. *Pocket Emergency Medicine*. Wolters Kluwer, 2015.

2. Mott, Timothy, and Kelly Latimer. "Prevention and Treatment of Drowning." *American Family Physician*, 1 Apr. 2016, www.aafp.org/afp/2016/0401/p576.html.

3. "Altitude Sickness: Symptoms, Diagnosis, Treatment & Prevention." *Cleveland Clinic*, my.clevelandclinic.org/health/diseases/15111-altitude-sickness.

4. K;, Kottusch P;Tillmann M;Püschel. "[Survival Time without Food and Drink]." *Archiv Fur Kriminologie*, U.S. National Library of Medicine, 2009, pubmed.ncbi.nlm.nih.gov/20069776/.

5. Silver, Natalie. "How Long Can You Live Without Food? Effects of Starvation." *Healthline*, Healthline Media, 29 Mar. 2019, www.healthline.com/health/food-nutrition/how-long-can-you-live-without-food.

6. Weiss, Thomas C. "What Happens When We Starve? Phases of Starvation." *Disabled World*, Disabled World, 2 Dec. 2020, www.disabled-world.com/fitness/starving.php.

7. Titi-Lartey, Owuraku A. "Marasmus." *StatPearls [Internet].*, U.S. National Library of Medicine, 20 June 2021, www.ncbi.nlm.nih.gov/books/NBK559224/.

8. WE, Roediger. "Metabolic Basis of Starvation Diarrhoea: Implications for Treatment." *Lancet (London, England)*, U.S. National Library of Medicine, 1986, pubmed.ncbi.nlm.nih.gov/2871346/#:~:text=A%20major%20component%20of%20starvation,energy%20to%20control%20absorption%20effectively.

9. Vandergriendt, Carly. "Everything You Should Know about Refeeding Syndrome." *Healthline*, Healthline Media, 6 Jan. 2020, www.healthline.com/health/refeeding-syndrome#symptoms   www.ncbi.nlm.nih.gov/pmc/articles/PMC2776367/.

CHAPTER 19: CONSCIOUSNESS AND COMA

1. Tindall, Suzie C. "Level of Consciousness." *Clinical Methods: The History, Physical, and Laboratory Examinations. 3rd Edition.*, U.S. National Library of Medicine, 1 Jan. 1990, www.ncbi.nlm.nih.gov/books/NBK380/#:~:text=Lethargy%20 consists%20of%20severe%20drowsiness,then%20drift%20back%20to%20 sleep.&text=Stupor%20means%20that%20only%20vigorous,back%20to%20 the%20unresponsive%20state.

2. Rajajee, Venkatakrishna. "Management of Acute Moderate and Severe Traumatic Brain Injury." *UpToDate*, 22 May 2021, www.uptodate.com/contents/ management-of-acute-moderate-and-severe-traumatic-brain-injury?search=trau matic+brain+injury+prognosis&source=search_result&selectedTitle=1~150&u sage_type=default&display_rank=1#H28.

3. Dennis, Bradley, et al. "Pentobarbital Treatment Guidelines for Severe Traumatic Brain Injury." *Division of Trauma and Critical Care*, Vanderbilt University, Nov. 2018, 6. www.vumc.org/trauma-and-scc/sites/default/files/public_files/ Protocols/Pentobarb%20Coma%20PMG.pdf.

4. Muhlhofer, Wolfgang G, et al. "Duration of Therapeutic Coma and Outcome of Refractory Status Epilepticus." *Epilepsia*, U.S. National Library of Medicine, May 2019, www.ncbi.nlm.nih.gov/pmc/articles/PMC6571024/.

5. Sutter, Raoul, et al. "Mortality and Recovery FROM Refractory Status Epilepticus in the Intensive Care UNIT: A 7-YEAR Observational Study." *Wiley Online Library*, John Wiley & Sons, Ltd, 7 Jan. 2013, onlinelibrary.wiley.com/ doi/10.1111/epi.12064.

6. Alex D. Cooper, MD. "Functional and Cognitive Outcome in Prolonged Refractory Status Epilepticus." *Archives of Neurology*, JAMA Network, 1 Dec. 2009, jamanetwork.com/journals/jamaneurology/fullarticle/798711.

7. Bates, David. "The Prognosis of Medical Coma." *Journal of Neurology, Neurosurgery & Psychiatry*, BMJ Publishing Group Ltd, 1 Sept. 2001, jnnp.bmj.com/ content/71/suppl_1/i20.

8. "Coma and Persistent Vegetative State." *Harvard Health*, 25 Feb. 2020, www.health. harvard.edu/diseases-and-conditions/coma-and-persistent-vegetative-state.

9. Maiese, Kenneth. "Vegetative State and Minimally Conscious State - Neurologic Disorders." *Merck Manuals Professional Edition*, Merck Manuals, Sept. 2020, www.merckmanuals.com/profes-

sional/neurologic-disorders/coma-and-impaired-consciousness/vegetative-state-and-minimally-conscious-state.

10. Maiese, Kenneth. "Vegetative State - Brain, Spinal Cord, and Nerve Disorders." *Merck Manuals Consumer Version*, Merck Manuals, Sept. 2020, www.merckmanuals.com/home/brain,-spinal-cord,-and-nerve-disorders/coma-and-impaired-consciousness/vegetative-state#:~:text=After%205%20years%2C%20about%203,of%20the%20original%20brain%20damage.

11. "List of People Who Awoke from a Coma." *Wikipedia*, Wikimedia Foundation, 31 Oct. 2021, https://en.wikipedia.org/wiki/List_of_people_who_awoke_from_a_coma.

CHAPTER 20: VENTILATORS

1. Alvarado, Andrea C. "Endotracheal Tube Intubation Techniques." *Stat Pearls*. U.S. National Library of Medicine, 27 July 2021, https://www.ncbi.nlm.nih.gov/books/NBK560730/.

2. "PTSD Symptoms Common among ICU Survivors." *Johns Hopkins Medicine*. Baltimore, Maryland, 26 Feb. 2013, www.hopkinsmedicine.org/news/media/releases/ptsd_symptoms_common_among_icu_survivors.

3. Epstein, Scott, and Allan Walkey. "Initial Weaning Strategy in Mechanically Ventilated Adults." *UpToDate*, 6 Apr. 2021, www.uptodate.com/contents/initial-weaning-strategy-in-mechanically-ventilated-adults?search=ventilator+weaning&source=search_result&selectedTitle=1~150&usage_type=default&display_rank=1.

4. Epstein, Scott K. "Weaning from Mechanical Ventilation: Readiness Testing." *UpToDate*, 10 Aug. 2021, www.uptodate.com/contents/weaning-from-mechanical-ventilation-readiness-testing?search=ventilator+weaning&source=search_result&selectedTitle=2~150&usage_type=default&display_rank=2.

5. "What Are the Possible Complications of Prolonged Intubation Following Tracheostomy?" *Latest Medical News, Clinical Trials, Guidelines - Today on Medscape*, 12 Nov. 2019, www.medscape.com/answers/865068-32832/what-are-the-possible-complications-of-prolonged-intubation-following-.

6. "Living with a Tracheostomy." *American Thoracic Society*, American Journal of Respiratory Critical Care, 2016, 7. www.thoracic.org/patients/patient-resources/resources/tracheostomy-in-adults-2.pdf.

7. King, Angela C. "Long-Term Home Mechanical Ventilation in the United States." *American Association for Respiratory Care*, Respiratory Care, 1 June 2012, rc.rcjournal.com/content/57/6/921.

CHAPTER 21: DEATH & DYING

1. Young, Bryan. "Diagnosis of Brain Death." *UpToDate*, 21 Apr. 2021, www.uptodate.com/contents/diagnosis-of-brain-death?search=death&source=search_result&selectedTitle=1~150&usage_type=default&display_rank=1.

2. Marchand, Lucille R., et al. "Death Pronouncement: Survival Tips for Residents." *American Family Physician*, 1 July 1998, www.aafp.org/afp/1998/0701/p284.html.

3. Torke, Alexa, et. al. "CEASE: A Guide for Clinicians on How to Stop Resuscitation Efforts." *Annals of the American Thoracic Society*, 6 Feb. 2015, www.atsjournals.org/doi/full/10.1513/AnnalsATS.201412-552PS.

4. Jain, Samay, and Michael DeGeorgia. "Brain Death: Associated Reflexes and Automatisms." *Neurocritical Care*, 2005, deqefw538d79t.cloudfront.net/api/file/3kaX5wPcTuPlwkBQwhAZ?cache=true.

5. Yasinski, Emma, et al. "Autopsy Rates Were Falling for YEARS. THEN Covid-19 Came along." *Undark Magazine*, 21 Oct. 2020, undark.org/2020/10/21/covid-19-autopsies/.

6. Dillon, Stephanie R. "Death and Kinetics." *Chemistry for Liberal Studies - Forensic Academy*, www.chem.fsu.edu/chemlab/chm1020c/Lecture%208/02.php.

7. Puiu, Tibi. "How Long Can a Person Remain Conscious after Being Decapitated?" *ZME Science*, 8 Oct. 2013, www.zmescience.com/research/decapitation-consciousness-042323/.

8. Roach, Mary. *Stiff: The Curious Lives of Human Cadavers*. W.W. Norton & Co., 2003.

9. Gerbis, Nicholas. "What Exactly Do They Do During an Autopsy?" *LiveScience*, Purch, 26 Aug. 2010, https://www.livescience.com/32789-forensic-pathologist-perform-autopsy-csi-effect.html#:~:text=Throughout%20the%20autopsy%2C%20the%20pathologist,and%20in%20recorded%20verbal%20notes.&text=If%20a%20complete%20internal%20examination,(if%20necessary)%20the%20brain.

Q&A

1. "How to Make a Tourniquet." *First CARE Provider*, First CARE Provider, 16 Feb. 2018, https://firstcareprovider.org/blog/tk-how-to.

2. Agabegi, Steven S., et al. *Step-up to Medicine*. Third ed., Wolters Kluwer, 2014.

3. Kellner, Charles H. "Speed of Response to ECT." *Psychiatric Times,* vol. 27, no. 5, 1 May 2010, https://doi.org/https://www.psychiatrictimes.com/view/speed-response-ect.

4. "Brain Injury and Sexual Issues." *Brain Injury and Sexual Issues - Better Health Channel,* https://www.betterhealth.vic.gov.au/health/conditionsandtreatments/brain-injury-and-sexual-issues.

5. Cotton, Simon. "Tetrodotoxin." *Chemistry World*, Chemistry World, 29 Jan. 2020, https://www.chemistryworld.com/podcasts/tetrodotoxin/3005972.article.

6. Jansen, Suze A, et al. "Grayanotoxin Poisoning: 'Mad Honey Disease' and Beyond." *Cardiovascular Toxicology*, Humana Press Inc, Sept. 2012, https://www.ncbi.nlm.nih.gov/pmc/articles/PMC3404272/.

7. Kupfer, David J, et al. "Catatonia." *Diagnostic and Statistical Manual of Mental Disorders: DSM-5,* American Psychiatric Association, Arlington, VA, 2017, pp. 119–120.

8. Girgis, Linda. "Top 14 Most Evil Doctors of the Last Two Centuries." *Physician's Weekly*, 25 Oct. 2019, https://www.physiciansweekly.com/top-14-most-evil-doctors-of-the-last-two-centuries.

9. Theobald, Brianna. "The Native American Women Who Fought Mass Sterilization." *Time*, Time, 5 Dec. 2019, https://time.com/5737080/native-american-sterilization-history/.

10. Dickerson, Caitlin, et al. "Immigrants Say They Were Pressured into Unneeded Surgeries." *The New York Times*, The New York Times, 29 Sept. 2020, https://www.nytimes.com/2020/09/29/us/ice-hysterectomies-surgeries-georgia.html.

11. Tikkanen, Roosa, and Melinda K Abrams. "U.S. Health Care from a Global Perspective, 2019: Higher Spending, Worse Outcomes?" *U.S. Health Care from a Global Perspective, 2019 | Commonwealth Fund*, The Commonwealth Fund, 30 Jan. 2020, https://www.commonwealthfund.org/publications/issue-briefs/2020/jan/us-health-care-global-perspective-2019.

12. Himmelstein, David U., et al. "Medical Bankruptcy: Still Common despite the Affordable Care Act." *American Journal of Public Health*, vol. 109, no. 3, 2019, pp. 431–433., doi:10.2105/ajph.2018.304901.

13. Finegold, Kenneth, et al. "Trends in the US Uninsured Population 2010-2020." Assistant Secretary for Planning and Evaluation: Office of Health Policy. 11 Feb 2021. https://aspe.hhs.gov/sites/default/files/private/pdf/265041/trends-in-the-us-uninsured.pdf

14. Tanne, Janice Hopkins. "More than 26,000 Americans Die Each Year Because of Lack of Health Insurance." *BMJ (Clinical Research Ed.)*, BMJ Publishing Group Ltd., 19 Apr. 2008, https://www.ncbi.nlm.nih.gov/pmc/articles/PMC2323087/.

15. Assistant Secretary for Public Affairs (ASPA). "New HHS Data Show More Americans than Ever Have Health Coverage through the Affordable Care Act." *HHS.gov*, 8 June 2021, https://www.hhs.gov/about/news/2021/06/05/new-hhs-data-show-more-americans-than-ever-have-health-coverage-through-affordable-care-act.html.

VOLUME 2 COMING SOON!

In *Volume 2: Illness & Injury*, you'll learn:

- Causes of chest pain other than the Hollywood Heart Attack
- Repercussions of traumatic brain and spinal cord injuries
- How to avoid cancersploitation
- The Deadly Dozen of traumatic chest injuries
- Myths vs. facts about suicide
- How bullets wreak havoc on the body
- What amnesia *really* looks like
- And more!

SNEAK PEEK AT VOLUME 2: ILLNESS & INJURY

BREAKING DOWN THE CLICHÉ: COUGH OF DEATH

Coughs into handkerchief in first act

Dies of terrible disease in the third act

A COUGH IS KIND OF LIKE the medical equivalent of Chekhov's gun, especially if your character is coughing up blood. In some ways, this cliché works; there are plenty of horrific diseases that present with a chronic cough. Lung cancer, metastatic cancer, tuberculosis, heart failure, sarcoidosis, fibrotic lung disease, and Chronic Obstructive Pulmonary Disease (COPD) are a few causes of chronic cough that could legitimately kill your character.

But there's also a lot of coughs that aren't fatal. Colds, asthma, acid reflux, and seasonal allergies are some of the most common causes of chronic coughs. You'd be hard pressed to kill your character with any of those.

The other thing wrong with this cliché is that coughs are not generally the first sign of a chronic or fatal disease. A mild fever–for no apparent reason–is often the first sign that your character has a blood cancer, like leukemia or lymphoma. Unexplained weight loss is often the first sign of other forms of cancer, as well as many chronic diseases like inflammatory bowel disease (Crohn's Disease & Ulcerative colitis), Celiac disease, HIV/AIDS, dementia, diabetes, and even depression.

If you want to foreshadow that your character is going to battle an illness, go beyond the chronic cough. Once you've decided what that illness is, look up the initial presenting symptoms. Find the vaguest one (usually weight loss or fever) and sprinkle that into your story. You can still have all the foreshadowing but avoid the cliché of coughing up blood into a handkerchief.

Ingram Content Group UK Ltd.
Milton Keynes UK
UKHW050914290323
419346UK00007B/50